VOICES OF THE AMERICAS

Traditional Music and Dance From North, South,
and Central America, and the Caribbean

A Concert and Cassette Series
Produced by the World Music Institute

Edited by Ray Allen

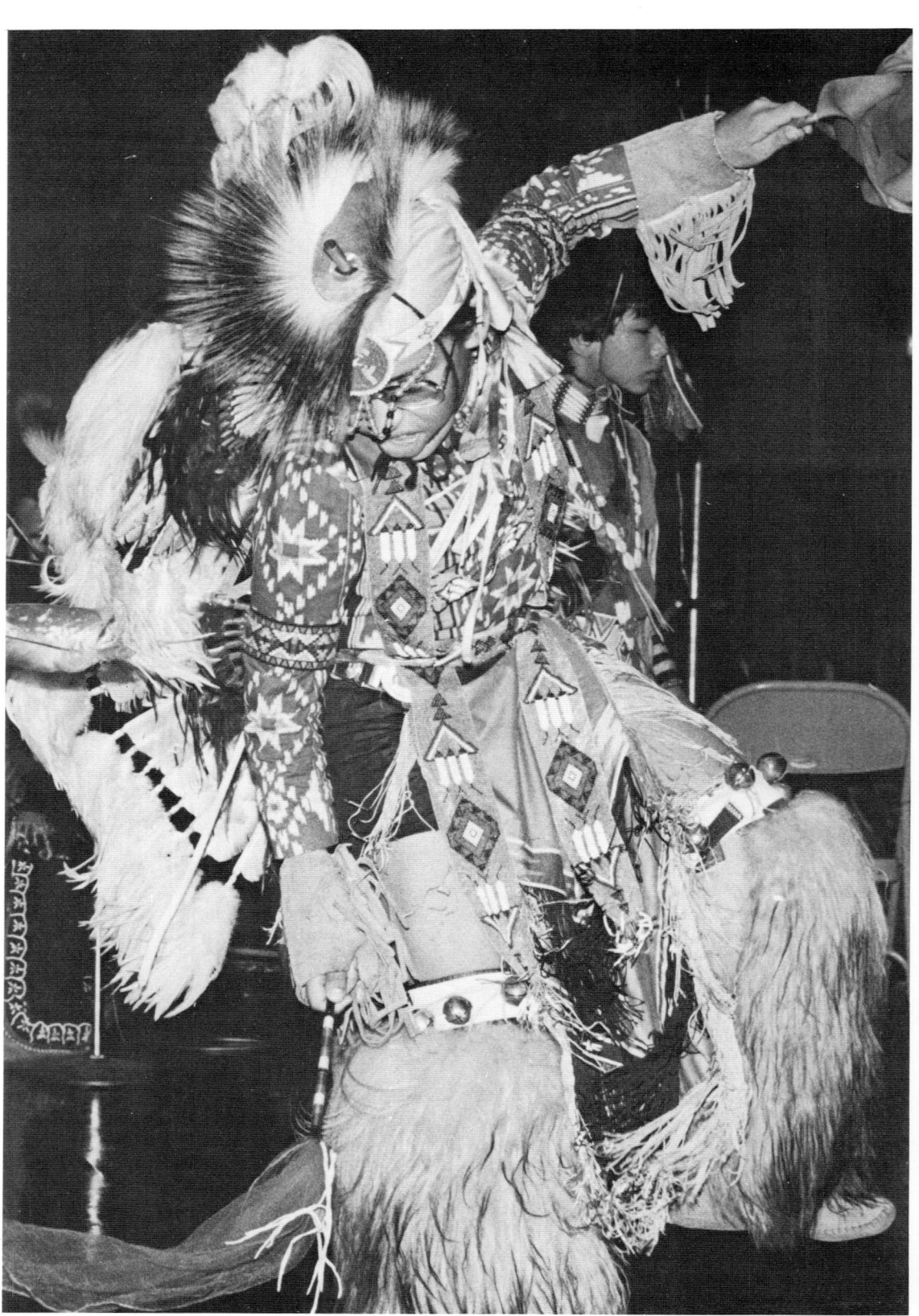
Standing Arrow Singers and Dancers.

Project Director: Robert Browning
Book Editor: Ray Allen
Design and Layout: Isabel Soffer

World Music Institute Staff:
Robert Browning — Executive Director
Ray Allen — Director of Research and Education
Bar Biszick — Production Manager
Isabel Soffer — Administrative Assistant
Helene Browning — Director of Promotion and Publicity

The World Music Institute is a not-for-profit organization founded to research and present the finest in traditional and contemporary music from around the world. Current programs include concerts of contemporary and traditional American music, non-Western classical music and dance by visiting artists, and traditional and contemporary folk music and dance from Africa, Asia, Europe and Latin America. WMI encourages and supports musicians from immigrant communities and collaborates with organizations that have similar goals. Other projects include the production of cassettes, radio programs, and booklets focusing on various aspects of world music. WMI also maintains an archive of concert and field recordings, and carries for sale a wide selection of cassettes and records of music from around the world.

Voices of the Americas is funded by the Folk Arts Program of the National Endowment for the Arts, the New York State Council on the Arts, and New York Council for the Humanities, and Friends of the World Music Institute.

All photographs by Robert H. Browning unless otherwise specified.

ISBN Number 0-945017-00-6
Library of Congress Number 87-051358

©World Music Institute, 1988
109 W. 27th Street
New York, NY 10001

This booklet is dedicated in memory of Manuel Vásquez and Sady Courville whose contributions to folk music of the Americas will be greatly missed but not forgotten.

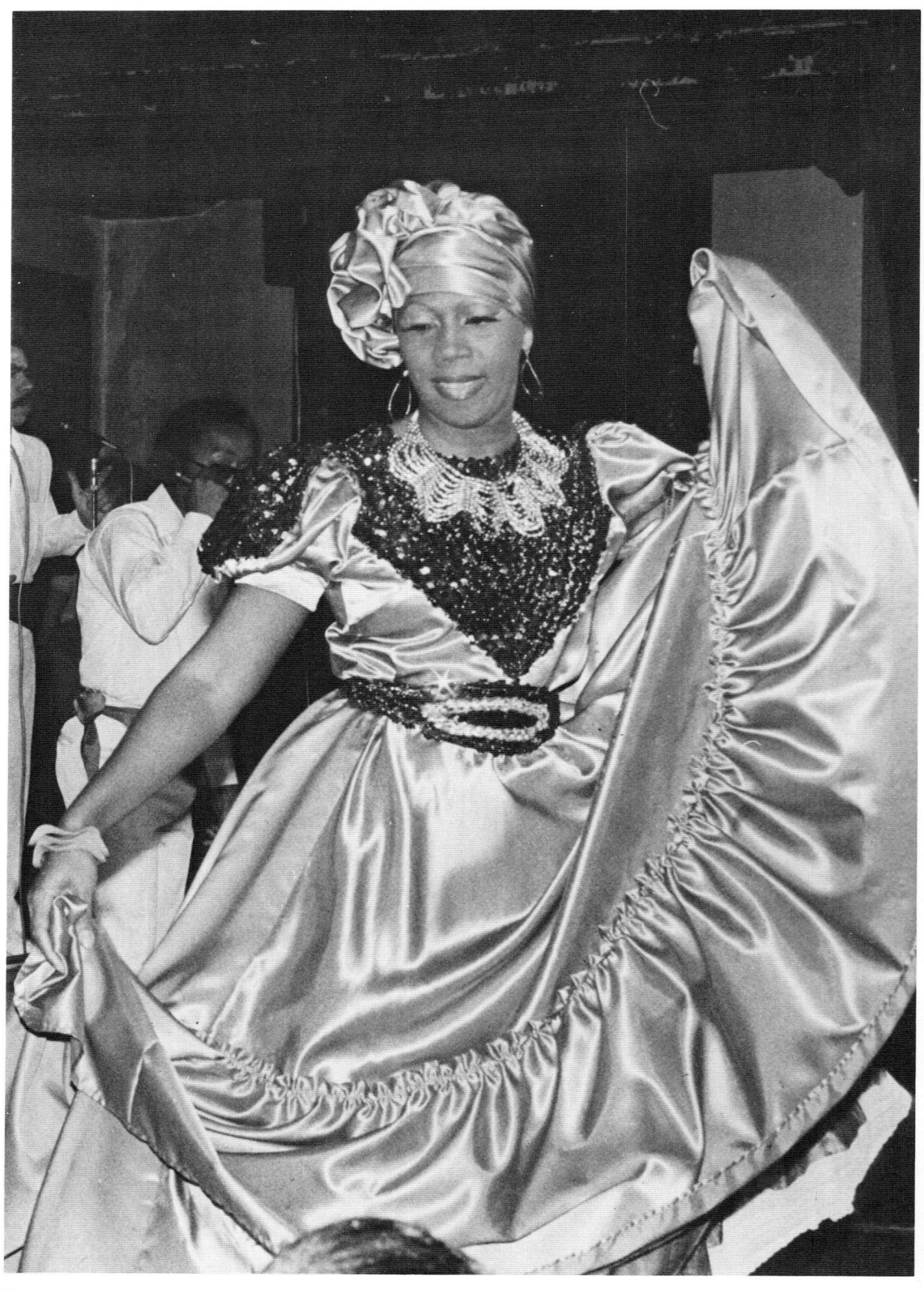

Xiomara Rodriguez with Orlando Puntilla Rios y Nueva Generacion.

CONTENTS

Forward	Robert Browning	6
Introduction	Ray Allen	7
Native American Music	David P. McAllester	9
Roots of the Blues	Peter B. Lowry	13
Early American Country Music	Kip Lornell	17
Spiritual Entertainment: African-American Gospel Music in New York City	Ray Allen	21
Puerto Rican and Cuban Musical Expression in New York	Roberta Singer and Robert Friedman	25
Cajun Music: A Louisiana French Tradition	Barry Jean Ancelet	33
Taking Spirit Time: The Vodoun Sounds of Haiti	Frisner Augustin and Lois Wilcken	37
Mexican Traditions: The Son Jarocho	Daniel Sheehy	41
Music of the Peruvian Highlands	Thomas Turino	43
Concert List		47
Biographies		49
Discography		59

Foreword by Robert H. Browning

Voices of the Americas is a multi-faceted project which grew out of a series of concerts of traditional music from North, South and Central America and the Caribbean presented by the World Music Institute in the winter and spring of 1986. The series took place at Washington Square Church in the heart of New York's Greenwich Village, a venue long associated with community-based events. Drawing on older rural and more recent urban traditions, the series featured both secular and sacred music. From live recordings of these concerts a set of 8 audio cassettes and an 8-part radio series were produced. This booklet is intended both as a companion to the cassette and radio series and as an introduction to some of the most widespread and influential music traditions of the Americas.

Voices of the Americas does not pretend to cover more than a fraction of the musical genres practiced by the diverse nations, communities and ethnic groups of the American continent. Since our resources were limited, we concentrated on North American traditions with Latin American and Caribbean traditions represented by immigrant communities living in the United States. The rich and varied traditions of Brazil, the English-speaking Caribbean and most of Central America will have to be left to a later series as will those of the more recent immigrant communities from Asia, the Middle East and southern Europe.

In an era of mass communication and homogenized popular culture, it is refreshing to discover that so many communities throughout the Americas have retained the unique character of their cultural heritage.

Indeed the recent interest shown by popular North American and European musicians in vernacular music, particularly that of Africa, the Caribbean and Latin America, has helped to regenerate pride in traditional music and dance within those communities. At the same time, it has kindled interest in a far wider audience often enabling musicians to earn a living by performing and teaching outside their communities. We hope that in some small way this project will continue the process of building a wider appreciation of the many musical traditions that have provided a source for so much of today's mainstream music, theater and dance.

I would like to take this opportunity to thank all those who helped to make this project possible: the Folk Arts programs of the National Endowment for the Arts, the New York State Council on the Arts and the New York Council for the Humanities which provided funding; the folklorists and ethnomusicologists who provided consultation and the essays for this booklet; Collegium Sound for providing sound reinforcement and recording the concerts; and the many volunteers and Friends of the World Music Institute who helped out at the concerts.

Special thanks to: John Baskind, Rita Calderon, Everett Chasen, Steve Cooper, Rebekah Foster, Erwin Frankel, Nancy Gross Bob Haddad, Glen Hinson, Barbara Jacksier Fran Lipman, Vicki Leota, Martha Lorantos Khalil Omkar, Laurie Russell, Robin Schiffman Don Wade and crew, Al Zucker, Martha Morriso and the staff of the Washington Square Church

Introduction by Ray Allen

Surveying the following articles and listening to the selections presented on the accompanying cassette series reveals an incredible depth, richness and diversity of musical expression. Despite centuries of slavery and colonialism, the persistence of political oppression and economic disparity, the social upheaval caused by industrialization and urbanization, and competition from mass media, community-based music continues to thrive and evolve throughout the Americas. Often referred to as "folk," "ethnic," or "vernacular," these styles exist outside the confines of the established Western high art tradition, and only on occasion are they authentically represented through the mass and popular media. Nevertheless, such vernacular musical expressions play vital roles in the lives of millions of North, Central, and South Americans, and during the past hundred years have left an indelible imprint on the so-called "high" and "popular" arts.

A number of important themes emerge upon closer examination of the essays and recordings. Perhaps the most significant of these is the concept of syncretism, a process by which musical elements of two or more distinct cultural styles are fused together to create a new, third style that retains elements of its predecessors, yet is unique. Syncretism has played a particularly crucial role in the New World, where European, African, and Amerindian musics have blended for centuries. While European and Native American peoples have mixed elements of their music cultures in various parts of Latin America, as Tom Turino describes in his essay on the High Andes traditions, the most vivid forms of syncretism appear as the result of the merger of European and African styles, particularly in the Caribbean and southern United States. For example, the Puerto Rican *bomba* and *plena* music discussed by Roberta Singer and Richard Friedman emerged from the fusion of Hispanic melody and verse/chorus song structure with West African elements of polyrhythm, improvisation, and call and response singing. Similarly, the Cuban *Santeria* music they describe, as well as the Haitian Vodoun ritual explored by Lois Wilcken and Frisner Augustin, exhibit the clear mixing of European and African worship and music traditions. African-American gospel music, the subject of my contribution to this volume, reflects the merger of European choral harmony with African rhythms, vocal timbre, improvisation, and body movement.

A second central issue is the effect of mass media, particularly the recording industry and radio, on vernacular musical traditions. Although traditional folklorists have long speculated that the electronic media would lead to the homogenization and eventual demise of regional folk styles, this has not always been the case. As Christopher Lornell and Peter Lowery point out in their respective essays on Euro-American country and African-American blues, the early radio and records helped preserve and spread traditional styles, often leading to further blending and the emergence of new syncretized forms. For example, the southwestern swing music performed by Junior Daugherty and the Chicago-style blues of Cary Bell evolved with the assistance of radio and recordings. Further, a number of older traditional styles—blues, early country, and various Afro-Caribbean expressions—eventually formed the foundation of the contemporary rock, soul, Latin, and country music that dominates the popular recording industry and radio/television airways today.

The concept of self-conscious revitalization has played a key role in various American music cultures, particularly during the past thirty years. In many areas of the New World, industrialization, urban migration, and immigration have threatened to eradicate traditional ways of life, including musical practices. In response to these pressures, younger (often educated, urban-based, and middle class) members of various ethnic communities have attempted to revive and revitalize older rural styles they feared were on the verge of extinction. For instance, as Tom Turino aptly reveals, young urban Peruvians have become outstanding exponents of what was once a traditional Amerindian mountain style. Barry Ancelot points to a similar phenomenon in southwestern Louisiana, where young Cajun players have revived the traditional styles from the early decades of this century. The pan-Indian Pow-Wows, described by David McAllester, reflect a similar impulse, as young urban Native Americans attempt to keep alive aspects of their traditional culture. Young Afro-Caribbean groups residing in New York

City, such as Los Pleneros De La 21, La Troupe Makandal, and Nueva Generacion exhibit elements of revitalization, as they strive to preserve the music, dance, and worship traditions of their native countries which are no longer widely practiced.

Finally, it must be underscored that the music represented in this booklet and cassette series is not played solely for the purpose of formal artistic or entertainment value—the primary function ascribed to Western and other "art" musics of the world. While aesthetic enjoyment is unquestionably important, this is only one of the multiple social functions served by vernacular musics. Within local and neighborhood settings, music performances such as the Saturday night blues, country, or Cajun dance provide occasions for community members to come together to socialize, strengthen communal bonds, and experience solidarity. *Bomba*, *plena*, certain blues and country songs, and Mexican *sones* often serve as vehicles for historical and social commentary and on occasion reflect thinly veiled protest. Other expressions—gospel, *santeria*, Vodoun, Andean fiesta styles, and Native American ceremonial forms—are tied to religious rituals and festivals, and reveal deep-seated views of the universe and Man's relation to nature and the spiritual world. Be they sacred or secular, many such styles serve ultimately as markers of ethnic identity and pride, reminding participants of their common historical roots and shared experiences. In doing so, vernacular musical expressions simultaneously reflect and support the cultural diversity of the Americas, and will undoubtedly continue to exert a significant influence in all spheres of social, political, and spiritual life for some time to come.

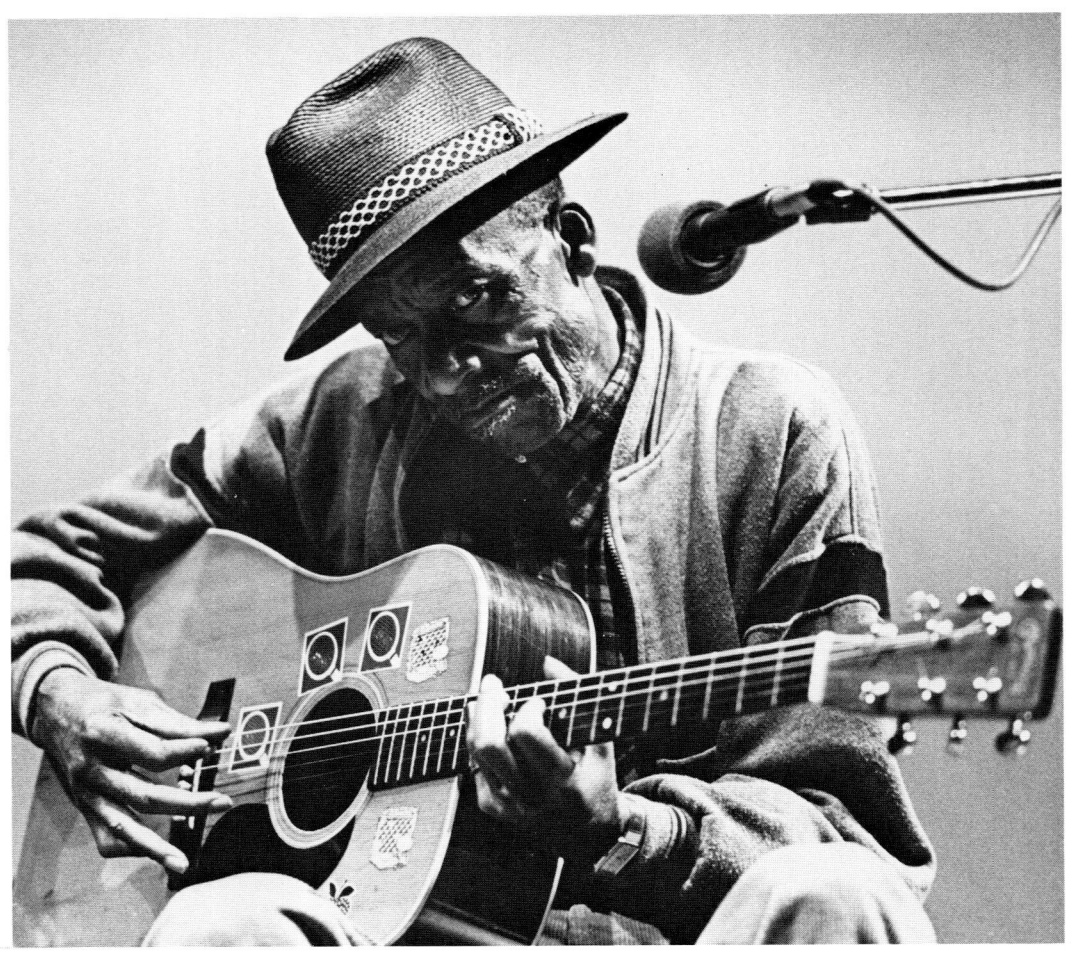

James Son Thomas.

Native American Music by David P. McAllester

Many "Native Americans" use that name for American Indians as a whole because their immigrant ancestors were the first to arrive in the New World 30,000 years ago, and did not come from India. In that incredible span of almost 2,000 generations the first Americans had time to develop customs, languages and musics with many elements that are unique among the cultures of the world.

Before I describe particular genres of this music I will point out some general features that characterize Native American music as a whole. I will be speaking, in this essay, in the "anthropological present" of about one hundred years ago when the traditional cultures were not yet greatly changed by European-American contact. Much of this description is still valid today. At the end, I will mention some of the new musics rising from the recent changes in Native American culture.

To begin with the general resemblances, *Native American music is almost entirely vocal:* except for flutes, whistles, and a few one-stringed fiddles, the musical instruments consist of a dazzling variety of drums and rattles used to accompany singing. *There are virtually no harmonies:* except for men and women singing an octave apart and a very rare use of parallel thirds, the singing and instrument playing are monophonic. *The singing style is robust:* songs tend to be loud, may have animal calls and other cries in them, and do not express sentiment by changes of speed and volume as most of ours do. The subtleties are in rhythm and melody where a high level of virtuosic art is displayed. *Song texts are usually short and vocabalic:* though some songs have texts epic in length, most Native American music has brief rhapsodic texts something like a Japanese haiku. These few phrases are often enclosed in vocables (untranslatable syllables) which make up the majority of the song. Many songs are entirely vocabalic. The translatable words usually refer to cosmic forces, deities, and sacred animals, birds, and places rather than personal feelings. *Most of the singing is by groups of men,* though there are personal and story-telling songs that are sung solo and men and women sing together in some kinds of social dance music. There are a few genres of song specifically for women. *The music expresses a world-view in which humankind is a cooperating part of nature:* the joyfully aggressive domination of nature by Euro-American culture is foreign to the traditional Native American ethos.

Music intersects every aspect of Native American life. There is music that accompanies each stage of the life cycle, from birth to death. There is music for nearly every activity: hunting, farming, canoeing, making war, visiting relatives, social dancing, and religious worship. This last category is so all-encompassing in the lives of Native Americans that they sometimes observe, "All our music is religious." Sacred song ranges from personal melodies learned in dreams to the songs of great ceremonials that take days to perform and may involve the efforts of hundreds of people.

I will begin my specific descriptions by sketching some of the best-known Native American religious festivals. "The Sun Dance" is so called by the Dakota. The Cheyenne call it "The New Life Lodge," and the Ponca call it "The Mystery Dance." It is a ceremony of the Plains tribes for the general good, to renew communion with the earth, sun, and winds, to ensure the health of the people and a plentiful supply of buffalo. The ritual includes the building of a sacred lodge, numerous offerings of food and other gifts to the forces of nature, and dancing, day after day, by individuals who have pledged their participation in return for help from the supernatural, such as the recovery of a sick child or a successful outcome in battle. In some tribes the sacrifices may include an offering by the dancers of their own flesh and suffering, a feature which has caused the U.S. Government, at times, to ban the ceremony. To the dancers the suffering is an indication of the seriousness of their gratitude for the gifts received from the deities and the natural world.

Through all this activity, which might go on for as long as eight days, there is music. The preparation for the ceremony includes many short songs by individual helpers about the correct way, learned in visions, to prepare sacred tobacco, bring in the first sacred pole of the Lodge, and other ritual acts. The dancing itself is to the thunder of a big drum played by several drummers in unison while a large chorus of men encourage the dancers with song after song, all in vocables. The dance songs are in a regular double meter and are typical of Plains singing: the voices soar up to a high, sometimes falsetto beginning, then make wide leaps downward and come to rest on the base note or tonic. They are made up of three or four short phrases and can be repeated as often as the singers wish. The vocal style is loud, tense, and pulsating. At intervals the drummers and dancers rest while officials of the ceremony sing prayer songs in freer rhythms than those needed for dancing. The Sun Dance, in its full performance, is a religious drama symbolizing the growth of vegetation and animal life, and also reminding the people of famous warriors and their battles.

"The Iroquois Midwinter Festival" reflects a different kind of celebration and renewal. At the New Year, the people of the great confederacy of the Six Nations bring together a number of dances and other ceremonial acts with the principal stress on thanksgiving. Some of the most important constituents are the Great Feather Dance, the visits of the False Faces (masked deities), the Bowl Game, and the confession of wrong-doing.

The singing with these events often begins with high calls ending in a downward glide, and follows a more undulating melodic line than the downward plunge of the Plains. There may be marked changes in speed in different sections of the song. A special feature among the Iroquois and other Eastern Woodlands tribes is responsorial singing. In the Quiver Dance, for instance, the leader introduces a series of short phrases like "Howiyo, howiyo!" which the other singers repeat, alternating with the leader phrase by phrase. The vocal style is like the forthright tone of European folk-singing. The phrases are longer and there are more of them in a song than in most Plains music.

The Iroquois have an unusual number of social dances, more than thirty, usually in a dignified, circular processional form. Many have names that indicate the Iroquois closeness to the natural world around them: Fish Dance, Robin Dance, Green Corn Dance, Duck Dance.

The Southwestern "Navajo Ceremonialism" is the most elaborate ceremonialism on the continent. There are more than twenty great healing chants that may take as long as nine days in performance and which contain thousands of lines of epic poetry based on a Creation Myth as complex as that of the Greeks. In addition there are uncounted shorter rites for healing, divining, and protection. The famous sandpaintings, of which several hundred have been recorded, portray episodes in the story of a particular ceremony. The performance of the long chants also includes prayers, sometimes dance, and, hour after hour, songs.

The songs are led by the medicine man (Navajo, *hatááli*—"singer") backed by all who know the melodies or can join in the choruses. They depict heroes going to the underworld, the sky, or other distant places in search of supernatural power to cure illness. The origin of the universe, the creatures in it, and the social customs of humankind are all explained. The powerful, buoyant singing in the ceremonies alternates between chanted narrative and more melodic choruses. Often built on the limited scale of the open triad and usually employing only two note values, the songs are miracles of shifting rhythms and subtle variations. The chanting is usually indoors and only for the ears of the initiated, but there is public dancing accompanied by singing as tense, highpitched and melodic as that of the Plains.

The formalized exchange of gifts is a widespread Native American custom, often as part of a ceremony. Its most complex expression was the "Potlatch" of the rich fishing communities of the Northwest coast. At the birth, coming of age, or death of an important individual a great feast would be held in which property would be given away or destroyed in overpowering demonstrations of wealth. Sometimes slaves would be killed or even the house of the host burned down in a kind of aggressive conspicuous consumption. The wealthiest guests at the feast had to equal such displays in return feasts, or acknowledge defeat in the social competition.

The many songs of the Potlatch were the private property of individuals or families, like everything else in Northwest Coast society. Many of the songs were sad evocations of the memory of a deceased member of the family and caused the singers and relatives to weep. Others were boastful accounts of the greatness of important families. They sometimes would rise in key as much as a third in the course of the song.

This kind of personal content is rare in other Native American music. Potlatch songs are remembered and owned today and are still sung at more modest celebrations, still called "Potlatches."

Snakes are honored all through the Southwest, perhaps in a vestige of the cult of the Plumed Serpent in Mexico. The most dramatic form taken by this reverence is in the "Hopi Snake Dances" in the mesa towns of western Arizona. The Snake and Antelope clans cooperate in prayer and ritual asking their brothers, the snakes, to take word to the gods in the underworld of the need for rain. In the public part of this ceremony the snakes are brought into the central plaza of the village and "danced" in a sacred circle, each with a pair of attendants. One holds the snake in his mouth, supported on either side with his hands, and the other strokes the snake's head with a feather to keep its attention away from his partner's face. After the dance the snakes are released in the four directions of the compass to carry out their mission.

The music for the various aspects of the ritual is deep and resonant, long and complex in melodic line, starts high and levels out on the tonic at the end. A special feature of Pueblo singing is sudden pauses, or brief shifts into triple meter, after long sections in rapid double rhythms. The words of the songs mention, over and over, clouds, rain, frogs, dragonflies, and other references to the water that is so scarce in this arid country.

In the late nineteenth century when Native American resistance to the encroachments of the white man was in its last stages, various religious movements and practices such as the "Ghost Dance" sprang up to accomplish what armed defense had failed to do. A prophet named Wovoka, in Nevada, had a vision of Jesus returning to help remove the invaders and bring back the buffalo. Word of the vision spread across the Plains along with a dance that led to visions of the next world. There, recently deceased relatives assured the visionaries of better times to come. The dance was a slow, ecstatic circling to plaintive, almost hymn-like songs in which each phrase was sung twice in the style of Paiute and other music of the Great Basin and Plateau country of Nevada and Utah. The music with its paired phrases, limited range, and quiet appeal was in marked contrast to the intense, vaulting stanzas of the traditional music of the Plains. This was the first of the pan-tribal Native American musics where a new musical form moved widely across the boundaries of tribal communities. A few old people still remember the Ghost Dance songs they heard from their grandparents, but the religion failed when the Messiah did not appear. The Native Americans had to learn to coexist with the vast numbers of new Americans who had flooded into their country.

From ancient origins among the Aztecs, "Peyote religions" using the peyote plant to induce visions came north towards the end of the 19th century and replaced the Ghost Dance religion of the Plains. Christian and traditional Native American elements have become commingled in the ritual. Prayers and songs are addressed to God and Jesus as well as Father Peyote; sobriety and the work ethic are important in the philosophy of what has become incorporated as the Native American Church. The night-long meetings are held in tipis, feather fans are used to draw the fragrant cedar incense to the participants, and the downward movement of the songs remind one, also, of the Plains. But the water-drum, the use of the open triad in many of the melodies as the basic scale and the frequent restriction to only two note values suggest a Navajo-Apache influence. The membership has spread pan-tribally and continues to grow: Native Americans feel that the Peyote Church is very much their own and includes Christianity and all other religions under one God and the teaching of Father Peyote. The new religion spread first in the Plains but now has thousands of members among the Navajos, too. There are meetings on the West Coast and in Canada: the pan-tribal movement has become international.

A number of other new musical traditions have been adapted by Native Americans during this century. A new and very lively spread of a traditional music to Native American communities all over the country is that of the Powwow. What were once war dance or Grass Dance songs of the Plains are now sung from coast to coast at social gatherings which feature a revival of Native costumes, give-away ceremonies, foods, and song and dance contests for cash prizes. Non-Native Americans, especially boys and young men in Scout troops, make superb costumes and tipis and learn the songs and dances well enough to compete seriously. Round dances are another feature of powwows; here men and women move about in a big circle, together. The musical style is that of the Plains, described above and the texts are usually entirely vocabalic.

Hymn singing is, of course, a new music of great importance to the many Native Americans who have joined various Christian denominations. Often the hymns have the slow meter and open harmonies of the Sacred Harp singing of Alabama and Georgia. Gospel and Gospel Rock are becoming increasingly popular.

Native Americans take a special delight in Country and Western music. There are also Native American urban Rock groups like "Redbone," "XIT," and "Jim Pepper." "Mr. Indian and Time," under the leadership of Eugene Beyale, is a Rock group that uses the idiom in an Indian way. Their songs urge young Native Americans to learn from their old people and preserve their cultural identity.

There are new genres using guitars, flutes, or full orchestra along with the voice to convey a Native American message to the world at large. J. Paul Ortega, a Mescalero Apache, sings about friendship and compassion as Indian virtues we could all emulate. Buffy St. Marie, a Cree, has a mystical message: her "Moonshot" depicts astronauts arriving on the moon and finding Native Americans already there, welcoming them. Arlene Norchissey Williams, a Navajo, puts her religious insights into song, with full orchestra, offering to share the Native American feeling for Nature. Louis Ballard, Quawpaw composer, has written choral and orchestral works on Native American subjects.

These new musics coexist with the traditional musics, many of which have retained their vitality or gained a new importance in the current revival of Native American religious and philosophical values.

David McAllester is a distinguished Professor of Anthropology and Music at Wesleyan University. One of the world's foremost authorities on Native American musical traditions, he has published numerous books and articles on the subject, including the classic works Peyote Music, Enemy Way Music, *and* Myth of the Great Star Chant.

Further Readings:

McAllester, David P., *Peyote Music*, (Viking Fund Publications in Anthropology, New York, 1949).

Morgan, Lewis H., *League of the Ho-dé-no-sau-nee or Iroquois*, reprinted as *League of the Iroquois*, Corinth Books, N.Y., 1962

Powers, William K., *Oglala Religion*, (University of Nebraska Press, Lincoln, 1977).

Spencer, Robert F. and Jesse D. Jennings, et al., *The Native Americans*, (Harper and Row, N.Y., 1965).

Tooker, Elisabeth, "The League of the Iroquois: Its History, Politics, and Ritual," in *Handbook of North American Indians, Northeast*, Smithsonian Institution, Washington D.C., 1978, pp. 418-441.

Underhill, Ruth M., *Red Man's Religion*, (University of Chicago Press, Chicago, 1965).

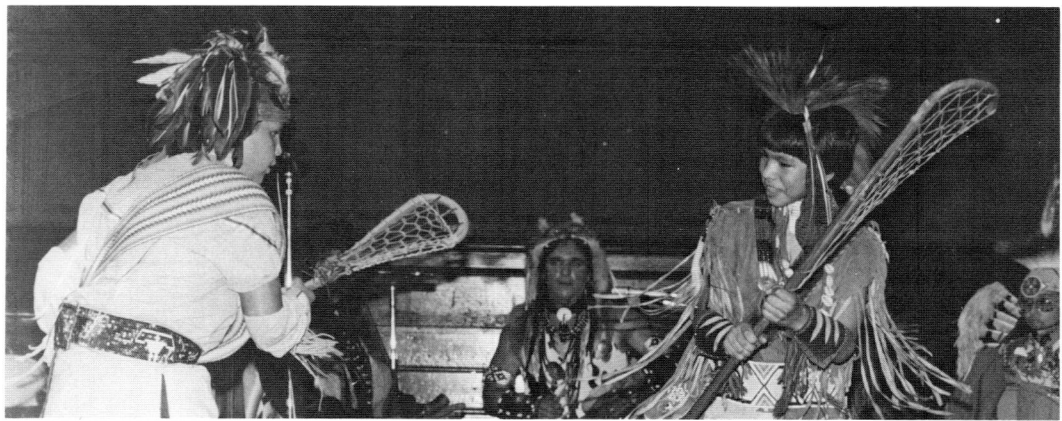

Standing Arrow Singers and Dancers performing a Mohawk Lacrosse Dance.

Roots of the Blues by Peter B. Lowry

Despite more than twenty-five years of scholarly attention, confusion and misunderstanding continue to surround the mysterious term "blues." This essay will try to uncomplicate things. In dealing with "blues" as a concept in African-American cultures, author Albert Murray makes an important separation of two of its meanings: "blues as music" and "blues as such." The latter concept is that of a feeling or attitude, of "having the blues," of insecurity and depression. The former concept embraces a type of music, and is to be the important focus here.

The music known as blues gathers into its definition a number of characteristics. Among them are musical notes that do not fit "properly" on the Western European chromatic scale ("blues notes"), a style of singing ("blues singing") and a predictable musical/lyrical structure ("blues verse"). Yet these attributes are not the sole way to classify—often songs are called blues, even when the above characteristics are lacking. This more generic, broader use of the term comes into play when the entire repertoire—including blues and non-blues material—of a performer generally perceived to be a "blues singer," is labelled "blues" for convenience sake. There are guidelines, but they are not etched in stone. Blues is often whatever it wants to be!

Blues music, as we know it, is definitely a 20th-century phenomenon. While its exact origins are unknown, interviews with older black musicians suggest that blues music appeared and spread throughout southern black communities sometime circa 1890-1910. Work songs, field hollers, country dance pieces, minstrel songs, and spirituals were among the numerous African-American sources from which the earliest blues evolved. While predominantly of black origins and fabrication, blues was also influenced by white American musical traditions. For example, the European narrative ballad helped give blues its lyrical structure, while the guitar (the primary blues instrument) came directly from middle class, European-American parlors. Such developments are not surprising, considering that black and white musical traditions in the southern United States have been in a state of constant interplay and interaction for many centuries.

This apparent rural southern form was codified somewhat in structure with the publication in the mid-teens of sheet music versions of blues songs—W.C. Handy is the best-known of those to publish. The form that predominated over time was characterized by a series of twelve-bar verses, each verse having an A,A,B rhyme scheme to its lyric. In the standard 4/4 rhythm of most American popular music, the twelve-bar verse is subdivided into three lines of four bars each. Generally lines one and two are lyrically the same, while the third line is different. That third line, however, usually rhymes with the first two and in some way resolves the intitial statement:

> My baby's gone, my baby's gone to stay. (A)
> Yes my baby's gone, that girl has gone to stay. (A)
> But the sun will shine in my back door some day. (B)

This "fixing" of the blues form, especially on sheet music, made it possible for large, organized groups of musicians to perform together. Smaller groups often "played" with the structure, and solo performers often honored the structure more by breaking it. Yet blues music has a form that is known and understood by all its players— only full understanding of such a structure permits moving away from that structure. The blues form became a common ground for black musicians throughout the country, rural or urban.

In the rural south, though, the music was not spread by sheet music (which unschooled musicians could not read), but by oral and aural means—initially from musician to musician directly, and later by means of the phonograph record. In a way similar to the impact of sheet music on blues musical *structure*, recordings had much to do with how a blues musical *performance* was perceived. In the rural south, a blues performance could be by a single person (often with a guitar or a piano for accompaniment), but generally there were more participants. For example, typical country bands often featured several guitars, and occasionally employed fiddle, mandolin, harmonica, and various home-made percussion devices. It all depended on who was available at that point in time, for most early southern blues performers were amateurs and did music "on-the-side". The impact of the music becoming preserved on recordings was rapid, and the effects were many. Records codified blues performance in the rural south in ways that sheet music could not—it took no notational literacy and it was immediate and repeatable.

The white record producers' aesthetic also came into play in the way recordings "fixed" aspects of blues performance. The black artists were asked to eliminate all spoken material from their pieces in the studio, and to use only the sung portions; that is how the producers viewed a "song". Also, the producers had difficulty with the normal loose-structured rural groups, so they preferred to record solo artists (or *rehearsed* small groups) if no formal band existed. After the Depression hit in 1929 and businesses in general were in difficulty, record companies cut back drastically on what they recorded. From 1920 to 1930, the first decade Afro-American musics were recorded commercially, the companies were willing to take chances on almost anything. After the Depression began, the surviving companies looked carefully at their sales figures and stuck with that which sold best. As a result, blues became the predominant form of secular black music to be sold to the black record-buying public. This, too, has had an effect on how blues "should be" performed, and is purely the result of economic conditions.

In the past, writers on black American music have taken "blues as music" and "blues as such" to be the same thing. This is not surprising, considering the racism and poverty that African-Americans have endured throughout their history. However, to suggest that blues is strictly a response to such oppressive conditions is too narrow an interpretation, for close analysis of blues lyrics reveals that overt complaint and protest are rarely expressed. Rather, blues songs are mainly about the difficulties of male/female relationships, while occasionally reflecting on such themes as travel, work, and the hardships of everyday life. The fact is there is a humorous, uplifting, even optimistic dimension to blues, particularly when performed in social gatherings where community members gather to eat, drink, socialize, and dance. In such settings rural African-Americans created their own expressions of entertainment to provide emotional release and strengthen communal bonds, and that is what blues music is really about.

If there is one important thing to remember about blues music, it is that it was and is mainly for dancing, the weekend blow-out! In their spare time, American blacks created many musics—some for religious purposes and others for secular celebration. There has been a tradition of "Saturday night" for just as long as there has been one of "Sunday morning". Before the turn of the century, blacks used fiddles, the banjo, drums, fifes, and other instruments that they could make for Saturday night music. At the turn of the century the country frolic had some form of string-band (using fiddle, mandolin, banjo, guitar, bass, etc.) playing for organized "set" dancing such as square, line or circle dances. Blues groups replaced string-bands at house parties by the 1920s, later were the primary music of southern juke joints through the 1950s, and are still a localized factor in black clubs in many urban centers today. Blues remains a music for celebration on a Saturday night in many black American communities—north *and* south. In the past there have been different ways of approaching and playing this musical genre in different geographical regions of the country. Some have fallen away in black culture, some have been maintained, and some have grown and expanded and changed over time.

If one looks at blues music as preserved and presented on phonograph records, it is possible to subdivide it into three general regions—southwest, south central, and southeast—that are stylistic categories as well as geographic ones. The three labels are rather loose in nature (especially the south central), but this perspective holds up well through the early post-war era. After that time, most of the regional differences were submerged as one homogenized style came to the fore commercially, one that had its roots in the southwestern modes.

Blues of the southwestern states (Texas, Oklahoma, western Louisiana and Arkansas, and, later, California) seems, from recorded evidence, to be blues of great rhythmic subtlety and swing. This is true of the jazz styles that came out of this region as well. In the blues, there is a rapidly articulated melodic line, single notes more often than chords, that has an understated rhythm. The lines played by the guitar are an extension or response to the vocal or melody of the song. The first major artist of the region from the standpoint of commercial success and influence on others was Blind Lemon Jefferson. In a sequence of historical figures over time, Jefferson was followed by Lonnie Johnson, and the tradition was extended even more by T-Bone Walker. It is the last-mentioned who essentially "began" the present-day homogenization in blues performances now concretized through the success of B.B. King.

The south central region (Mississippi, eastern Arkansas and Louisiana, western Alabama and Tennessee) is the one that eludes any single stylistic generalization, especially in the early days of recording. There have been attempts by scholars to do so in the past (the term "Delta blues" is one most often seen in print), attempts that do not hold through the region at all. In trying to set characteristics, such music is often described as being harshly chordal, percussive and hypnotic, even crude, a music with dense rhythms and raspy vocal style. This may be true of some musicians' work from parts of the south central area like Charley Patton or Bukka White. The work of other musicians, however, does not pigeonhole at all well. Certainly the plaintive modal stylings of Skip James, the near-ragtime finger-picking of Robert Wilkins, or the songster approach of Mississippi John Hurt bear this out. And there are many more besides these three. The patchwork of styles that made up the south central blues remained as a localized phenomenon for quite a long time, with only a few spreading beyond their locale. As blacks moved to urban centers, first Memphis and then St. Louis, Detroit, and Chicago, a sort of common ground developed that was shared by musicians as they migrated. People like Muddy Waters or Elmore James epitomized that change, updating their older style and smoothing out the rough edges. Later urban developments came out of the B.B. King method, one that had its start in Memphis, but was very much a synthesis of *many* blues styles.

Blues in the southeast (Georgia, the Carolinas, Virginia, northern Florida, eastern Tennessee, Kentucky, and Alabama) has been an interesting phenomenon, for the general picture developed from phonograph recordings shows a remarkably homogeneous style throughout the region by the time of the Depression. The music is highly syncopated, and is centered on a finger-picked guitar style that has a very strong ragtime basis. Beyond the ragtime factor, that is also a strong input from white old-time or "hillbilly" music. The most important names in this region, again from the standpoint of record sales and influence, were Blind Blake, Josh White, Buddy Moss, and Blind Boy Fuller. Later musicians like Brownie McGhee or Tarheel Slim attempted to update the music, but without commercial success in the black record-buying marketplace. As a major style of black music on a commercial scale, the southeastern blues faded out in the fifties, becoming once again a local phenomenon.

To return to the subject of phonograph recordings, the discs allowed a budding performer to hear other than local musicians in developing a style. In fact it allowed blues styles to leap geographical limits, and, by the thirties, the regional styles were being slowly affected by those from outside. This was especially true for black musicians living in cities. Their local stylistic network was often gone as rural neighbors went separate ways, and so the 12-bar AAB blues structure became the common link between musicians from different rural localities. It allowed for "musical communication" between them as they played more as professionals for audiences that were *not* necessarily of identical cultural backgrounds. But communicate they did, both with each other *and* their audience...and as a result, blues styles changed.

As has been indicated, the main *national* impact on blues performances came out of the southwest's single-note, melodic style. Aaron "T-Bone" Walker updated this approach and made it accessible in two ways. First he used an electrically amplified guitar that made it a true lead instrument, and, second, he used a jazz-like band to back his singing and playing. Since this was close to what was happening in black popular music in general (jazz combos and singers), he made blues easily accessible to that audience. His records sold nationwide and had an important impact on an up-and-coming musician in the Memphis area named Riley B. King. Mississippi-born B.B. King took Walker's music, that of some local blues artists (like his uncle Bukka White), and added to that a bit of the jazz of Belgian gypsy guitarist Django Reinhardt and alto sax player Louis Jordan. From that mixture he formed his own horn-like guitar style that he used to front a small jump combo. In addition to his legato, single-note guitar, King added a vocal style that came right out of the black church. It is Mr. King's approach to blues music that has had an impact on *all* blues singers and guitarists, from all parts of the country since his first hit records of 1953!

After the war, records were not just something to play at home or on a juke box. About 1949 some southern radio stations took notice of the large black audience and began to program shows aimed at it. Both recordings and "live" performances on radio helped spread blues in general, and the King approach in particular. And that exposed younger white musicians to blues, which eventually resulted in the rock & roll explosion of the 1950s. Early rock & roll was another melding, this time of blues and boogie-woogie with swing and country and western.

Today, blues music exists as both a commercial and local form. No longer is its audience totally black; in fact, most of the audience for the music may be white, and much of it is not even American! There is still a "national" approach to the music in the King mold, as well as more localized approachs (such as exists in Chicago), although that is not untouched by Mr. King. The earlier, pre-war regional blues styles became, at best, highly localized forms of black music, as rural bluesman lost any possible national audience to the urban blues performers who dominated the record and radio industries in the post-war years. A few of the former—James "Son" Thomas, John Holeman, John Jackson, Phil Wiggins and John Cephas—found a new, non-black audience for their traditional styles on the folk festival circuit. For most of the elder musicians, however, the old rural blues is only a memory.

Post-war urban blues, coupled with the later soul music, continues to hold considerable appeal for select black and white American audiences. In cities such as Chicago, Detroit, Memphis, Los Angeles, and Houston, some form of an updated blues scene exists. Artists such as B.B. King, Albert King, Bobby Bland, Little Milton, Albert Collins, Magic Slim, and Carey and Lurrie Bell are successful today. Blues still exerts an enduring influence on contemporary American popular music, as B.B. King's approach to blues guitar has now become the point-of-reference for most rock and pop instrumentalists. It has been a long lived and tough critter, this music for a good-time Saturday night!

Peter Lowry has done extensive field research among African-American blues musicians in the southeastern United States. He is presently a Ph.D. candidate in the University of Pennsylvania's Department of Folklore and Folklife.

Further Readings:

Bastin, Bruce. *Red River Blues: The Blues Tradition in the Southeast* (Urbana: University of Chicago Press, 1986).

Keil, Charles. *Urban Blues* (Urbana: University of Chicago Press, 1966).

Oakley, Giles. *The Devil's Music: A History of the Blues* (New York: Harcourt, Brace, Jovanovich, 1976).

Murray, Albert. *Stomping the Blues* (New York: Random House, 1976).

Palmer, Robert. *Deep Blues* (New York: Penguin Books, 1981).

Early American Country Music by Kip Lornell

Country music, like blues, evolved from several distinct styles of primarily American music. Defining this music is a difficult task because it includes so many genres, such as Cajun, western swing, and honkytonk, with strong regional ties or cultural connotations. Furthermore, country music has clear links to such diverse traditions as minstrel shows, British and native American balladry, Scots and Irish fiddle tunes, and shape-note singing. The presence of black Americans is felt in the influence of blues, and the pervasiveness of an African instrument, the banjo.

If Nathan Abshire's Cajun accordion, the swing orchestra of Bob Wills and his Texas Playboys, and Merle Travis' Kentucky finger-picking all qualify as country music, how does one pinpoint **the** geographic source for this music? As another uniquely American idiom, jazz, country music is undeniably the product of multi-genesis. Moreover, there is no doubt that the single most important region for country music has been the Appalachian highlands. This often rugged and beautiful section stretches from southern New York to northern Alabama, and has long been both its wellspring and well. These mountains have spawned important, diverse, and influential performers like the Carter Family, Patsy Cline, Loretta Lynn, Ernest V. "Pop" Stoneman, Dolly Parton, Roy Hall and the Blue Ridge Entertainers, the Stanley Brothers, Wade Mainer, and the Statler Brothers.

The prominence of Appalachian performers in country music is obviously not a recent phenomenon. Many of the prolific country recording artists from the 1920s, including Fiddlin' John Carson, Henry Whitter, the Carter Family, Al Hopkins and the Bucklebusters, and Gid Tanner and the Skillet Lickers are closely associated with Appalachia. Not surprisingly the first commercial country record, which was released in 1923, was Carson's "The Old Hen Cackles and the Rooster's Going to Crow" and "Little Old Log Cabin in the Lane." Similarly, most of the early radio stations that were broadcasting in the southeastern United States, such as WSB in Atlanta, Washington, D.C.'s WRC, and WDBJ in Roanoke, Virginia, featured regularly scheduled live programs by local country musicians. These broadcasts were particularly important because they brought the music of many different performers into hundreds of thousands of homes across the entire country.

Of course, many styles of country music existed well before the 1920s. "Old-time" fiddle tunes like "Sally Anne" and "Old Joe Clark" were being performed before the turn of century, and Reconstruction minstrel show stages often featured small stringbands as part of their presentations. In fact, many such traditional expressions played important roles in the social lives of the Appalachian people. Fiddlers provided lively dance music for community gatherings, balladeers and songsters entertained friends and family in domestic settings, and sacred singers added an essential musical component to worship services.

The commercialization and nationwide dissemination of country music by fledgling radio stations and the revitalized record industry provide us with its first aural documentation. Because many of these radio stations, and nearly all of the commercial record companies were based in the East, the prominence of Appalachian performers is understandable. Radio stations were built across the entire eastern seaboard and utilized the musical talent around them. This resulted in radio performances by early country performers John Carson, Gid Tanner and his Skillett Lickers, Riley Puckett, and other Atlanta-based artists over WSB as early as 1922.

Record companies, on the other hand, operated in the North, especially New York City. By the mid-1920s, record company executives were beginning to comprehend the commercial potential of country music, and slowly began to build a network of talent scouts and record dealers in the South to supply them with musicians. Because of the Appalachian's well-deserved reputation for music, many representatives looked towards the Southeast as a source for "hillbilly talent."

Through the use of newspaper ads, radio announcements, and word of mouth, it was easy to locate country musicians in the Appalachian highlands. Some musicians were transported to northern studios, but many were recorded on portable equipment setup in cities such as Knoxville and Bristol, Tennessee, Asheville, North Carolina, and, most often, Atlanta, Georgia.

During the first major period of country music recording, 1923-1930, scores of Appalachian musicians were documented by commercial record companies.

These musicians encompassed a large number of genres and styles. Some performed older British ballads such as "Barbara Allen" or "The Farmer's Curst Wife," or a native American ballad like "The Wreck of the Old 97." Ballads, which told often sad or moralizing stories, were often sung a cappella, but most early hillbilly recording artists recast them in the format of a small stringband. Although these "stories in song" used to be commonly found across the United States, the southern Appalachian highlands remain a stronghold for such ballads.

Appalachia also has had a reputation for physical and cultural isolation, which partially explains the continued strength of and interest in ballads. Nonetheless, by the 1920s the industrial revolution had come to these mountains in the form of highways, railroads, textile and furniture factories, and radio. The newer, sentimental songs written by Tin Pan Alley writers at the turn of the century were easily accepted by mountain musicians. Thus it was not unusual for an Appalachian singer's repertoire to include "On The Baggage Coach Ahead" or "The Yellow Rose of Texas," in addition to ballads.

The Carter Family is perhaps the single most influential country music recording group from this period. Their mixture of ballads, religious songs, folk songs, and blues is also emblematic of early country music from the Appalachian highlands. This trio started off as a family group that performed in and around Scott County, in southwestern Virginia. Their major break came in 1927 when they successfully auditioned for the Victor Company and shortly thereafter recorded at the field session in nearby Bristol. Their recordings sold well and launched them on a full-time professional career that lasted through World War II. In addition to their scores of recordings for Victor, Decca, and the American Record Company, the Carter Family performed over the radio and at numerous school houses throughout the southern Appalachians.

The Carter's are sometimes called the "First Family of Country Music," an accolade in keeping with the status they earned in the 1920s and 1930s. It also speaks to the family orientation of early country music. Successful acts from the 1920s and 1930s, such as the Pickard Family and the Stoneman Family, underscore this observation. Country music was literally a family affair, and was used as an important social outlet.

Portions of families often got together to make music. By the middle 1930s brother duets had risen to country music prominence. This was when the Delmore Brothers from Alabama, and Kentucky's Charlie and Bill Monroe were being emulated by singers around the country. Their close-harmony singing and twin-guitar or guitar/mandolin work served as the model for later recording artists like the Morris Brothers and Roy and Jay Hugh Hall who lived in the mountains of western North Carolina.

It is impossible to talk about early country music without a brief mention of the influence of religious traditions. The majority of these musicians came from church backgrounds and have played sacred music. Two of the most prominent early recording groups, the Carter Family and Ernest V. Stoneman and his Dixie Mountaineers, explored both aspects of their repertoire. The religious music that so profoundly affected these pioneers basically stems from two roots: shape-note singing and the fervent tunes of the evangelical revival.

Like so many aspects of American life, the commercial country music industry was profoundly influenced by the Depression. Prior to 1930 the record industry documented all types of unknown talent, which resulted in records by delightful and obscure groups like the Wise String Orchestra (Vocalion), the Arkansas Barefoot Boys (Okeh), and the Weems String Band (Columbia). The sour economy severely limited their interest in all but proven sellers like the Carter Family.

Another important trend in 1930s country music was an increasingly less regional and more homogeneous sound. This music was going "up-town," moving further away from its roots, and towards the popular sound of country swing and cowboy singers like Bob Wills, Milton Brown, Bob Boyd, and the Sons of the Pioneers. Their records sold well and their radio broadcasts affected musicians across the country. The entire country was caught in a western craze that affected clothing styles, movies, and books in addition to music.

This was true even in the most conservative sections of the Appalachian highlands. Cowboy tunes were being played by solo performers and stringbands throughout this area. In Roanoke, Virginia, for instance, local country radio artists from the mid-to-late 1930s sported names like the Wanderers of the Wasteland and the Dixie Playboys, and emulated their favorite western swing artists.

The nature of country radio was changing in other sections of the country as well. The most dramatic change came in the form of "border radio stations" based on the Mexican/American border that broadcast at powers that far exceeded the United States' 100,000 watt limit. Their night signals covered much of North America, and they often featured country music acts such as the Callahan Brothers, the Chuck Wagon Gang, and the Pickard Family.

The last major trend in country music before World War II was the development of bluegrass. With strong roots in the music of eastern Kentucky, the main progenitor of bluegrass was Bill Monroe. However, it quickly found a welcome home in the "Tri-State" section of western North Carolina, northeastern Tennessee, and southwestern Virginia. It could be argued that bluegrass is the result of multigenesis, and was simultaneously developed by several Tri-State bands. Certainly the late 1930s and early 1940s recordings by Byron Parker and His Hired Hands, Roy Hall and the Blue Ridge Entertainers, and the Morris Brothers lend credence to this line of thought.

For all practical purposes World War II marks the end of the early years of American country music. Certainly the war itself had a profound impact on country music by limiting the musicians' travel. And for a period in 1943 the musicians' union dispute stopped all recording. The immediate postwar decade was characterized by a larger number of radio station seeking new formats, Nashville's rise to prominence as recording center, and the virtual explosion of small, independent record companies. These factors altered the very nature and distinctly southern flavor of country music. Today's less regional, often bland commercial country music can be heard on juke boxes, in bars, and over the radio from Portland, Maine, to Portland, Oregon.

Despite the homogenization of country music, regional styles still exist, though they are all but ignored by major commercial record companies and radio stations. However, "old-time" string band music, traditional bluegrass, and ballad singing retain strong followings in certain areas of the South. These and other styles represent the continuation of grassroots American country music that is destined to remain an important part of our culture, and a source for the Nashville treadmill for many years hence.

Kip Lornell holds a Ph.D. in ethnomusicology and an M.A. in folklore, and has been researching, recording, and writing about American vernacular music and culture since 1969. Much of his work has been carried out through the Blue Ridge Institute of Ferrum College.

Further Readings:

Green, Douglas B., *Country Roots: The Origins of Country Music* (New York: Hawthorne, 1976).

Malone, Bill, *Country Music U.S.A.* (Austin, Texas: University of Texas Press, 1985).

Malone, Bill and Judith McCulloh, eds. *Stars of Country Music* (Urbana: Illinois; University of Illinois Press, 1977).

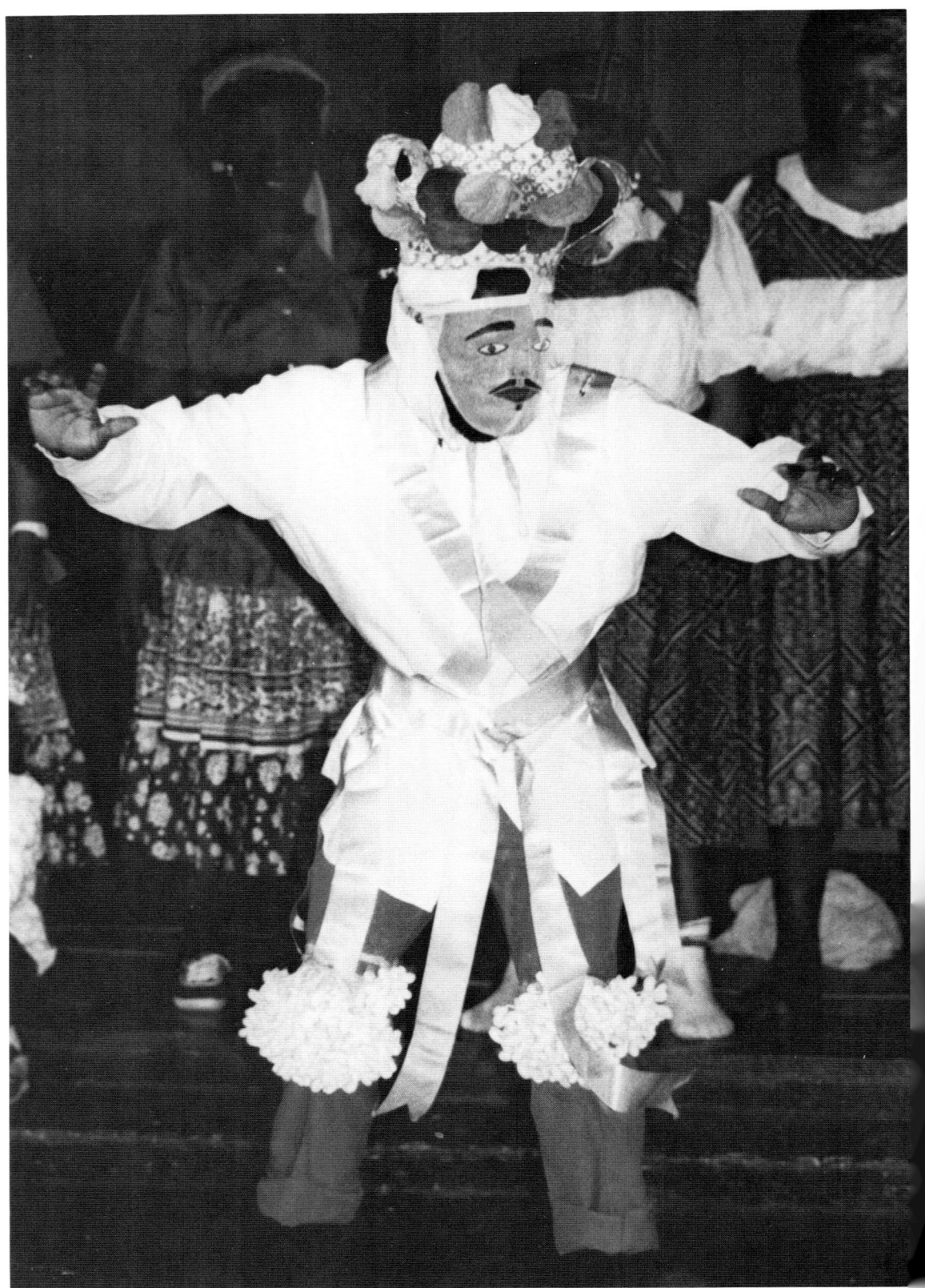
Garifuna Folk Dance Ensemble performing the *Wanaragua* or "John Canoe" masked dance.

Spiritual Entertainment: African-American Gospel Music in New York City by Ray Allen

"Gospel music is spiritual entertainment, and it is something that was given to black people by God," reflects David Steward, dynamic lead singer for the Wearyland Gospel Singers, one of New York City's premier gospel groups. "And the Bible tells you, make a joyful noise. So you see it really is entertainment for spiritual people. You feel good, you have a good time in the name of the Lord, no matter where you are—in a church, a school, a theater, no matter where!"

Steward's comments summarize quite clearly the deeply felt sentiments shared by most African-American gospel singers. They see themselves as artists who provide aesthetic enjoyment and spiritual fortitude for their listeners, as their songs carry messages of Christian love, salvation, and the possibilities of liberation from the burdens of an often hostile world. Gospel singers have created one of America's most original and enduring musical expressions, and their story is only now beginning to be told.

While the term "gospel" in African-American music is usually used in reference to a style of sacred singing which emerged in northern and midwestern urban centers sometime around the late 1920s, the roots of this tradition reach back to the rural folk music of the South. The melismatic moans of the spiritual and folk hymn, the emotional fervor of the ring shout and song sermon, the pulsating rhythms of sanctified music, the tight harmonies of minstrel and black college quartets, and the syncopated licks of jazz and blues all contributed to the evolution of African-American gospel music. These southern folk expressions were brought north during the early decades of this century as part of the great migration of rural blacks who poured into urban centers in search of better economic opportunity and escape from the oppression of southern racism. Early gospel composers including C.A. Tindly of Philadelphia, Thomas Dorsey of Chicago, and W.H. Brewster of Memphis drew heavily on these older styles in shaping their music. The gospel sound that emerged—characterized by a basic call (leader) and response (chorus) structure, the use of driving, syncopated rhythms, and a highly emotive, improvised lead vocal—became the dominant form of African-American religious song from the 1930s on.

Fueled by an expanding radio and recording industry, gospel music rose to new commercial heights in the post-World War II years. Female soloists like Mahalia Jackson, Sallie Martin, and Roberta Martin, along with female harmony groups like the Ward Singers and Davis Sisters, carved out lucrative careers as touring and recording artists. Meanwhile the older male a cappella jubilee quartets began absorbing elements of the new gospel music into their performances. Lead singers Ira Tucker of the Dixie Hummingbirds, Rebert Harris of the Soul Stirrers, and Julius Cheeks of Nightingales worked their audiences into spirit-induced frenzies with a "hard gospel" style that often resembled ecstatic southern preaching.

By the 1960s it was choirs, and soloists backed by choirs, that began to dominate the commercial field of gospel. Some singers, most notably James Cleveland and Shirley Caesar, maintained a traditional, southern tone to their singing, complete with spirited testimonies and an emotional, shouting-style vocal. More recently, however, modernists like Al Green, Andre Crouch, and Edwin Hawkins have shaped a smoother-sounding style, known as "contemporary gospel." This music, which has become a dominant commercial force in the mid-1970s and into the 1980s, makes use of sophisticated musical arrangements and advanced studio techniques, and borrows freely from the stylistic elements of modern black pop music.

Today gospel music continues to flourish. As a multi-million dollar recording and entertainment business, gospel music has become a major form of mass-produced, black popular culture. In the local, non-commercial sphere, however, gospel thrives as an enduring statement of African-American community, faith, and aesthetic style. Every Sunday afternoon, in black communities across America, thousands of non-professional gospel soloists, groups, and choirs take to the floors of local churches and community centers, many of them singing for little or no monetary compensation. In performance these artists embody an aesthetic sensibility firmly based in the African-American tradition. Further, the ritualized atmosphere they create allows listeners to reaffirm their religious convictions through the shared experience of the Holy Spirit.

It is not surprising that New York City, which currently is home to the largest urban population of African-Americans in the United States, boasts a long legacy of outstanding gospel music. During the 1930s, jubilee and spiritual singing quartets like the Southernaires and the Selah Jubilee Singers gained national recognition through their recordings and radio broadcasts. New York's status as a recording and entertainment center prompted early gospel stars including Virginia's Golden Gate Quartet and the Norfolk Jazz and Jubilee Singers to relocate in the city. Two outstanding female vocalists of the early post-war era, Ernestine Washington and the Georgia Peach, also saw their careers come to fruition in New York City. In recent years the area has produced some of the country's most noteworthy choirs, including the New York and New Jersey Mass Choirs, Brooklyn's Institutional Radio Choir, and the Timothy Wright Concert Choir.

While these professional gospel artists have received a good deal of national attention, little is known about the local, non-commercial groups that form the backbone of New York's gospel community. Every Sunday, hundreds of these non-professional gospel choirs and groups perform in the neighborhood churches of Harlem, Bedford Stuyvesant, Jamaica, and the South Bronx. These performances vary significantly in size and quality, ranging from small, storefront church affairs to huge gospel extravaganzas held in large churches and theaters. The former may involve only one or two groups, while the latter often feature a dozen or more groups, often including one or two out-of-town acts. The money raised by local groups at such programs is often donated back to the sponsoring church, or goes toward the purchase of new uniforms, instruments, and travel expenses.

A wide variety of musical styles is exhibited in these programs. Large choirs singing older folk hymns and church songs as well as contemporary gospel arrangements are popular. However, it is the small performing ensembles—male, female, or mixed "groups" and "quartets"—which continue to be the mainstay of these local programs. A few have maintained the older, a cappella style of singing, which features tight, four-part harmonies and an accentuated, moving bass vocal. Most, however, use guitar, bass, drum, and keyboard accompaniment, and feature several lead vocalists who can shout the church with fast, "hard" songs, or soothe the listeners with the softer, "sweet" numbers. Post-war gospel compositions make up the bulk of these groups' repertoires, although most also feature a substantial number of older folk hymns, revival songs, and spirituals which have been rearranged in gospel style.

Gospel programs, which are usually held on Saturday evenings or on Sunday afternoons, take on many of the trappings of a Sunday morning church service. Both begin with a devotional service which usually consists of congregational singing, prayer, a scripture reading, and a period of personal testimony. While the Sunday morning service proceeds with the preacher and sermon taking center stage, in the gospel program it is the singers who deliver God's message through sung and chanted words.

The atmosphere of these gospel programs is fiercely competitive. Although groups no longer engage in official "song battles" as they did in the past, most readily admit they are attempting to outsing their competitors. Groups are greatly admired for their original and innovative song arrangements, and for their ability to perfectly balance, or "blend" their voices in tight harmony. Long hours are spent in weekly rehearsals, creating and refining these vocal arrangements, to assure that singers will not be accused of "copying behind" another group or recorded arrangement. Lead singers are expected to be able to "work" their congregations in order to "build the spiritual feeling." They accomplish this through a number of performance strategies including the prefacing of songs with lengthy chanted narratives and personal testimonies; shifting from a sung to a chanted/preached vocal delivery during improvisory "drive" or "gospel" sections of songs; switching lead singers in mid-song, or having two lead singers improvise together in a call and response fashion; and engaging in various dramatic gestures and movements such as acting out song lyrics or prancing up and down the aisles.

While such expressive behaviors are most certainly meant to demonstrate artistic competence and showmanship, they ultimately create an emotionally charged atmosphere which is conducive to bringing on the experience of the Holy Spirit. During a particularly moving performance, singers and congregation members may become overcome by the power of the Holy Ghost, and enter into trance-like states in which they shout, cry, chant in prophetic speech, run through the audience, or holy dance. During such periods of heightened physical and emotional awareness, some may actually reexperience the feeling of their original conversion experience, while others simply rejoice in the immediacy of the Almighty's presence. Thus, in its ritualized frame, community-based gospel music becomes more than simply Sunday afternoon entertainment. Through song, chanted testimony, and the Spirit-induced shout, gospel performance serves the dual role of reaffirming the faith of believers while bringing the Christian message to unsaved, potential converts.

In addition to religious concerns, a strong sense of southern identity often surfaces during gospel performance. New York City's African-American community has strong southern roots, as the vast majority of older gospel singers and churchgoers are southern-born migrants. In order to appeal to this crowd, certain gospel groups often identify themselves with their southern hometowns, even though they have lived in New York for years. The lyrics of songs and testimonies are rich with romantic imagery of the rural South, often urging listeners to go back to the "old-time" way of southern life when people worked hard, respected their families and elders, and practiced genuine Christian values in their everyday lives. These themes are contrasted to the dangers of northern, urban life—crime, drugs, prostitution, broken families, and the general decay of moral and religious values.

For many members of New York City's African-American community, ritualized gospel performance becomes a symbolic vehicle for the maintenance of southern religion, moral values, and identity. Particularly for older, southern-born individuals, gospel serves as a mechanism for combating the constant encroachment of urban, secular life; it reminds its participants who they are, where they came from, and how they can achieve ultimate triumph and liberation from the burdens of this world.

Today the so-called "contemporary gospel" sound, which has dominated the commercial industry in recent years, is making strong inroads in the local New York City scene. The younger, New-York-born performers and their audiences have become increasingly drawn to this style, which features a smoother approach to vocal and instrumental shadings, and lacks the fiery testimonies and evangelical tone of the older "traditional" gospel. Most younger groups and choirs, however, continue to take pride in their ability to sing both the traditional and contemporary styles, a versatility which allows them to reach congregations of all ages. This ability to simultaneously look forward and back—to constantly create innovative new forms based on older, traditional materials—appears to be a hallmark of African-American religious performance.

In New York City, and undoubtedly in dozens of other major urban centers, community-based gospel music continues to play a vital role in the lives of many African-Americans. Local gospel artists provide their communities with artistic enjoyment, spiritual strength, and a sense of historical identity. They help raise money for financially strapped churches and charitable causes, and their efforts often result in attracting new church members and bolstering church attendance. In performance they enter into the mysterious world where art and religion intersect, as they render the intellectual suppositions of fundamentalist Christianity emotionally convincing through the evocation of deep spiritual, moral, and aesthetic sentiments. Hence, in the words of singer David Steward, gospel music truly serves as "spiritual entertainment"—a dynamic artistic force which helps bind together a community of believers.

Ray Allen, currently Director of Research and Education at the World Music Institute, holds a Ph.D. from the University of Pennsylvania's Department of Folklore and Folklife. His dissertation research was based in New York City's African-American church community.

Further Readings

Helibut, Tony. *The Gospel Sound.* (New York: Anchor Books, 1985).

Broughton, Viv. *Black Gospel* (Dorset, England: Blanford Press, 1985).

Lawrence Levine. *Black Culture and Black Consciousness* (New York: Oxford University Press, 1977).

Southern, Eileen. *The Music of Black Americans* (New York: W.W. Norton and Company, 1983).

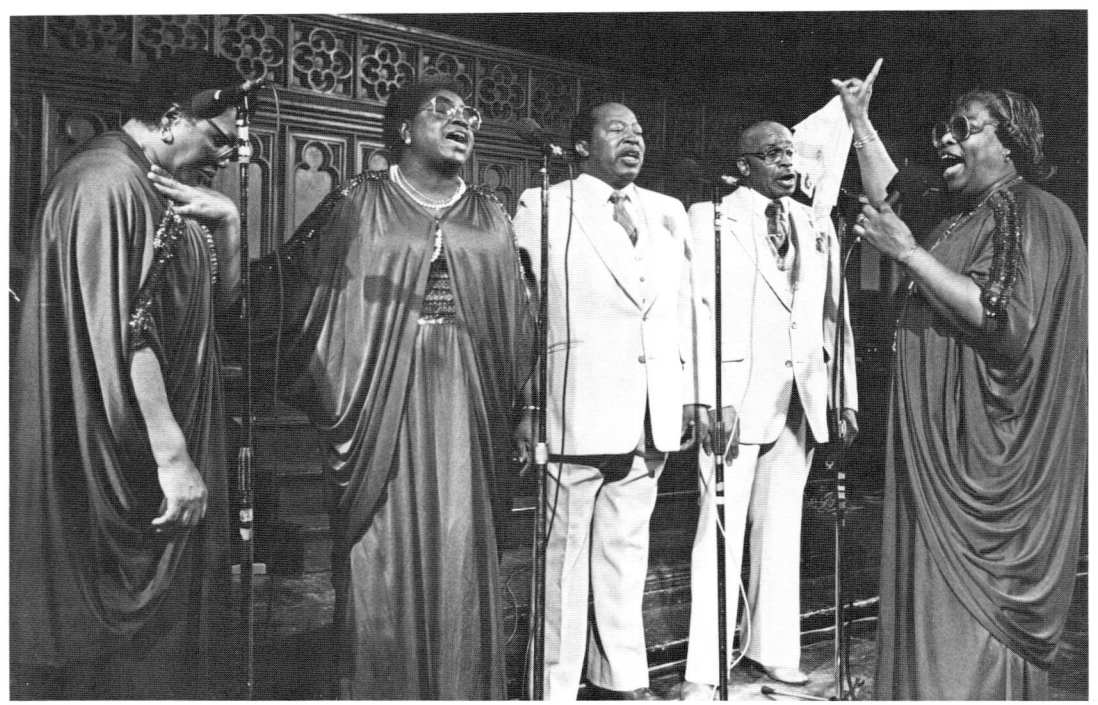

The Faithful Harmonizers led by Reverend Vernella Kelly.

Puerto Rican and Cuban Musical Expression in New York
by Roberta Singer and Robert Friedman

In New York the phrase "Latin music" has come to mean the up-tempo hot Latin dance-band sound currently known as *salsa*, but the history of Latin music in New York goes back further than the salsa industry. (*Salsa*, literally "sauce," is used to describe the feeling performers put into their music, like "savory," "spicy," "tangy." Thus playing *con salsa* means playing with soul.) Earlier in the century, Tin Pan Alley, Broadway, and Hollywood borrowed some of the music and dance forms of Mexico, Cuba, and Argentina and incorporated these elements to add "flavor" and a touch of "exoticism." The tango dance craze to which this thirst for exoticism gave rise lasted through the 1930s and spread throughout Europe as well as the United States. But the music was merely a Latin-flavored Tin Pan Alley stereotyped imitation. This was not the case with the Cuban rumba craze that swept the United States and the Continent at the start of the thirties. (*Rumba* music is known as *son* in Cuba. *Son* and *rumba* will be discussed below.) The craze was short-lived in Europe and everywhere in the United States except New York, where a sizable Latino community had begun to form in East Harlem. *El Barrio* (literally "the quarter"), as this community was known by its residents, created a second major audience for Latin music in New York. The first continued to flourish in the downtown and East Side nightclubs that catered to white audiences demanding Americanized versions of Latin music. The Latino audiences demanded the real thing, which they got in the uptown dance halls and nightclubs.

In 1898, after the Spanish-American War, Puerto Rico became a protectorate of the United States, and in 1917 the United States imposed citizenship upon the Puerto Rican people. With citizenship they were free to travel between the island and the mainland without the delays and restrictions faced by other immigrant groups. By this time the island's economy had experienced an agricultural industrialization as a result of North American investment. In the 1920s this industrialization began to decline and in the 1930s reached total collapse. Although it remained profitable to investors throughout the Depression, agricultural industrialization proved unable to provide a subsistence wage for the majority of the people. This economic upheaval gave rise to movement from the rural areas to the cities and in many cases from the cities to the mainland when work could not be obtained on the island.

Migration from the island to the mainland was significant in the 1920s and 1930s, but the factors that stimulated migration became sharply aggravated in the 1940s, when there was a shift from agriculture to industry, once again as a result of North American capital. This industrialization, however, could not absorb the growing labor pool. The demand for unskilled or semiskilled labor in industry and the service sector on the mainland, combined with unemployment on the island and the Puerto Rican government's encouragement of migration, resulted in massive migrations starting immediately after World War II. Two additional factors facilitated these migrations: the Puerto Rican government made an agreement with the Federal Aviation Administration to lower transportation rates between the island and the mainland, and large media campaigns on the island lauded the values of moving to the United States, which was depicted as the land of opportunity.

The massive migrations lasted until the end of the 1950s, and although there has been a decline in the numbers of migrants, the flow continues to the present. A factor of great importance is the constant contact that migrants and their children have maintained with their island home through frequent messages, letters, telephone calls, and visits.

While Puerto Rican migrants have settled in nearly every state, New York City has by far the greatest concentration. El Barrio was the first major Puerto Rican community in New York and remains the best-known, although it is no longer the largest.

In the late 1940s, people from the same town on the island began to form hometown social clubs. These clubs, named after the home towns (for example, Club Lares, Club Ponce), were intended to re-create the hometown environment. They also gave the members a means of coping with an alien environment, assisted the newcomer in adapting to life in the city, and provided a forum for the discussion of the problems of daily existence. The clubs were usually converted factory lofts decorated with artifacts, memorabilia, and photographs from home. They were family-oriented places where members could come together to socialize in a manner they had been used to on the island. The music performed in the clubs provided entertainment and also aided in creating a sense of the hometown. As a rule, the *cuarteto* sound of the *jíbaro* (rural dweller) dominated these settings.

Cuban migrations to New York, although significant, never reached the proportions of the Puerto Rican migrations. A primary factor was the stringent United States laws imposing a quota on the numbers of immigrants. Some Cubans managed to circumvent the quota system by going first to Puerto Rico and from there entering the United States, but this accounts for only a small number of Cuban immigrants.

The economic factors that stimulated migrations from Puerto Rico also existed in Cuba, but the economic problems of the *campesino* (farmer) and urban unskilled or semiskilled laborer were compounded by racial issues. The Spanish colonizers had transported African slaves to Cuba in much greater numbers than to Puerto Rico, hence the black population was sizable. Socioeconomic distinctions were made primarily along racial lines, relegating a disproportionate number of blacks to the lower strata. Black Cubans who came to the United States before the revolution of 1959 cite racism in Cuba as a strong factor in the decision to emigrate.

Aided by a relaxation in the laws, immigration patterns changed after the revolution. Before 1959 the majority of Cuban immigrants were from the lower classes, and of these a large percentage were black. Although some *campesinos* and urban dwellers (black and white) continued to enter the United States after 1959, a disproportionate number of immigrants came from the middle and upper socioeconomic strata. The new immigration was top-heavy with businessmen, intellectuals, and professionals.

Other Hispanic peoples have migrated to New York in significant numbers, although never in the same proportions as the Puerto Ricans. Immigrants from Cuba, the Dominican Republic, Panama, Colombia, and Venezuela, among others, settled in the areas established by the Puerto Ricans, but more often formed their own distinct communities. The Cubans, for example, are concentrated in the area west of Broadway and north on 133rd Street and in sections of Washington Heights.

Jíbaro Music Forms

Seis, aguinaldo, mapayé, and *danza* are Spanish-derived forms for solo voice and instrumental accompaniment. The *danza* is the only one that was written by composers in the Western art-music tradition and the only one that developed among the elite in the urban areas of Puerto Rico. Possible influences on the *danza* were the Cuban *habañera* and the European country dance. The *danza* had become popular all over the Caribbean in the nineteenth century and was performed by dance orchestras modeled after European salon traditions. The *danza* is the only form whose structure in sectionalized in the manner of European art music. The piece begins with an introduction (*paseo*), which is followed by a minimum of two contrasting sections, each of which is repeated. The number of contrasting sections is at the discretion of the composer. The Puerto Rican *danza* is distinguished from other Caribbean *danzas* by a distinctive rhythmic structure.

In the early nineteenth century, large plantations (*haciendas*) were formed as a result of the Spanish land grants, which gave one family control over large portions of land, much of which was already being worked independently by *jíbaros*. The hacienda system relegated the *jíbaro* to a position of subservience to the landowner (*hacendado*), making him a sharecropper. The *hacendados* perceived themselves as an aristocratic rather than agrarian class. They made frequent excursions from their country homes to the cities for a variety of reasons, including entertainment, which they sought in the salons. *Danzas* and other European-derived musical and dance forms were played in these places. Many *hacendados* also acquired pianos for their homes. The piano and the European-oriented music played on it were symbols that reinforced the *hacendados'* aristocratic pretensions. In addition, the *hacendados* invited orchestras from the cities to perform on special occasions at their haciendas. In this way the *jíbaros* came into contact with these musical forms, many of which they adapted to their own expressive styles. For the most part, forms such as the *danza* retained their structure but were adapted to the instruments of the *jíbaros:* guitar, *cuatro* (a small ten-stringed guitar-like instrument), *maracas* (a pair of rattles), and *güiro* (a scraped gourd). The word *cuarteto* refers to various combinations of these instruments and has come to symbolize the "typical" sound and repertoire of *jíbaro* music.

In addition to the adaptations of European art-music forms, the *jíbaros* possess a varied repertoire of traditional music. Forms such as the *seis, aguinaldo,* and *mapayé* are derived from music brought to the New World by the Spanish settlers.

The *seis* (literally "six") takes its name from a six-couple dance and refers to a variety of musical and dance forms, although not all *seises* are intended for dancing. The improvised texts of *seises* are often based on a *décima* (ten-line-stanza) structure, with each line consisting of six or eight syllables. This improvised stanzaic form, common throughout Latin America, is frequently incorporated into other forms of *jíbaro* music.

The *mapayé* is a form more popularly known as *le lo lai*, after the vocables sung at the beginnings of various verses. *Le lo lai* is characterized by a more varied harmonic structure than that of the other *seises* and is always in the minor mode. The texts of *le lo lai* are generally improvised around nostalgic themes of homeland, motherhood, nature, and idealized love, themes that characterize much of the *jíbaro* repertoire.

The *aguinaldo* differs from *danzas* and *seises* in that the former has come to be associated with a particular season. During Christmas, groups traveled from house to house singing *aguinaldos* and asking for small symbolic gifts such as food and drink. *Aguinaldo* texts, whose contents may be relilgious, secular, or a combination, are based on a *décima* structure.

With the migrations of *jíbaros* from the rural regions to the urban areas of Puerto Rico, the musical forms underwent a shift in emphasis. In the country, the *danza, seis, mapayé,* and *aguinaldo* were used for entertainment at all types of formal and informal gatherings. In the cities, special occasions such as weddings, baptisms, and holidays became the primary settings for these forms. *Jíbaro* musical expression in New York found its outlet in the hometown social clubs, where it again was used for informal entertainment as well as for special occasions. With the decline of the hometown social clubs in the 1960s, and the increasing popularity of *salsa*, *jíbaro* music is now played only at Christmas time and at folk festivals.

Bomba and Plena

Bomba and *plena* are the only distinctive African-derived musical and dance forms of Puerto Rico. They both developed in the coastal towns, where large communities of black workers gathered around the sugarcane mills. *Bomba* is an entertainment form and is generally performed at social gatherings. It is a couple dance in which the woman performs relatively fixed dance steps while her partner is free to exhibit his dancing skills. He dialogues with the "lead drummer," who rhythmically responds to his steps. The *bomba* ensemble consists of *fuá* (a pair of sticks struck on the side of a drum or some other hard resonant surface), which provides a fixed rhythmic pattern (time line) around which the other instruments are organized; one or two *buleadores* (low-pitched barrel-shaped drums), which provide a fixed supporting rhythm; and *subidor* (higher-pitched barrel-shaped drum), which plays changing rhythmic patterns within the rhythmic structure of the *buleadores* and *fuá*. (The terms *buleadore* and *subidor* refer not only to the names of the drums in the ensemble, but also to the drums' musical function. The *buleadore* is always a supporting drum, and the *subidor* is an improvisatory drum.) The specific manner in which these patterns are organized is regulated by the rhythmic nature of the song text and the movement of the male dancer. In addition to the *fuá, buleadore,* and *subidor,* maracas or a *güiro* may be included in the ensemble, increasing the rhythmic density and drive. A *campana* (cowbell) is optional and may substitute for or be used in addition to the *fuá*, reinforcing the time line. *Bomba* texts are usually on topical themes relating to everyday life in the community, such as social relationships, work, or historical events. They may also be spontaneous statements commenting on activities taking place in the performance. The musical form of *bomba* consists of alternation between solo singer and chorus in a call-and-response pattern. The soloist, having textual and melodic freedom, presents the main themes of the text, while the chorus is restricted to a fixed response.

Plena, although African-derived, incorporates more European musical elements than does *bomba*. *Plena* began as a street music, but it also moved into the bars and nightclubs where it came to be associated with night life. Although white and black musicians performed *plena*, the whites associated it more with slumming, but for blacks *plena* was a valid part of their musical heritage. *Plena* is a couple dance, but the dance is not an integral part of the event, as it is in *bomba*. The dialogue interaction between drummer and dancer that characterizes *bomba* is not found in *plena*. A typical *plena* ensemble consists of a number of percussion instruments including several *panderetas* (frame drums) and a *güiro* that provide fixed, interlocking rhythmic patterns. An additional *pandereta* improvises extended rhythmic passages that accent portions of the rhythmic structure of the text. Accordion and/or harmonica provide additional melodic embellishment, while a guitar is occasionally employed for harmonic accompaniment. *Plena* texts are on contemporary or historic events and are in a stanzaic verse-refrain structure.

In New York, *bomba* and *plena* have undergone certain transformations. Their use at informal social gatherings—and in the case of *plena*, in nightclubs—has sharply declined. However, their content is being reinterpreted in the salsa *conjunto* (small-group) format. Moreover, in recent years there has been a renewed interest in Afro-Puerto Rican cultural heritage among older and younger community musicians who are revitalizing *bomba* and *plena* traditional expressions.

Santería

An important form of musico-religious expression of Puerto Ricans and Cubans in New York derives from beliefs and practices of the Yoruba people of Nigeria and Dahomey in West Africa. The belief systems of the Yoruba and other African peoples were brought to the New World as a result of the slave trade. Voluntary organizations provided a means for these peoples to maintain their identity in the post-slavery period. From these organizations, which were known in Cuba as *cabildos,* the Yoruba-derived Lucumí and other religions and secret societies of African origin emerged. Lucumí beliefs are characterized by complex relationships among the forces of nature, concepts about the creation of the world, the pantheon of *orishas,* and man. Each *orisha* is associated with various myths, herbs, stones, colors, animals, and musical forms. An individual is devoted exclusively to one *orisha,* who may, during ritual events, possess his devotee. Once this is accomplished the *orisha* becomes actualized in human form and can interact with participants in the event. The philosophical foundation and organizing framework for these beliefs are centered in a system of divination known as Ifa.

Syncretism between Catholicism, as imposed by the Spaniards, and the African belief systems of the slaves resulted in certain superficial changes in Santería, the most common of which was overt acceptance of the symbols of Catholicism in an effort to mask Santería religious practices (e.g. saints' names were equated with *orishas*). This was necessitated by the attempts of the dominant political and religious structure in Cuba to force blacks to sever ties with their African heritage and thus gain greater control over them. Despite such superficial changes in Lucumí, adherents made a conscious attempt to maintain a close identification with Yoruba practices by using the Yoruba language in religious contexts and by observing the function the role of the *orishas*, musical practices, and numerous other aspects of their world view. However, two basic changes occurred in Cuba. Whereas in Africa each religious center was devoted to one *orisha,* and an individual's dedication to that *orisha* was determined mainly by lineage, the situation in the New World did not allow for an individual center to be committed to one *orisha.* Instead, each center paid homage to the entire pantheon.

The migrations of Cubans to New York City, both before and after the revolution, led to the establishment of religious centers in New York. The multi-ethnic character of the city is reflected in the religious centers. Membership now includes black and white North Americans as well as Cubans, Puerto Ricans, and other Latino groups.

Music functions in Santería as the central organizing feature of different events in the ceremony. *Igbodú* and *Eya Aranla* are separate events in the ceremony, and each serves a particular ritual purpose. The purpose of the *Igbodú* is to pay homage to the pantheon of *orishas* through a set liturgical sequence of rhythms known as *Orú del Igbodú*, which is performed on the *batá* while members stand in silent reverence. *Batá* is a drum family composed of three different-sized instruments, each of which is double-headed and hourglass in shape. They are held horizontally, with one hand on each membrane. The largest drum, *iyá*, communicates directly with the *orishas*, each of whom has his or her own identifying rhythms. The *iyá* also enters into musicolinguistic conversations with the *itótele*, the second-largest drum. *Okónkolo*, the smallest drum, plays a rhythmic pattern that changes when signaled to do so by the *iyá*.

The ritual purpose of the *Eya Aranla* is to facilitate communication between the *orishas* and the devotees. This is done through the *Orú del Eya Aranla*, a series of chants performed for each *orisha* by a lead singer (*akpwón*) and chorus (*ankori*) in a call-and-response pattern while the *batá* play corresponding rhythms. The *Orú* is performed to call the *orisha* into the ceremony. When called, the *orisha* manifests itself in human form through possession of individual devotees. In this way the *orisha* is now able to communicate directly with the participants.

Rumba

Rumba is the generic term for a group of African-derived Cuban musical and dance forms. Each form reflects a different degree of syncretism among African and Spanish linguistic, musical, and dance elements. Since slavery times *rumba* has provided a means for commentary on a wide range of issues, such as political and social events affecting the life of the community.

Three of the better-known forms of *rumba* are *guaguancó*, *yambú*, and *columbia*. The instrumental ensemble for *guaguancó* and *columbia* is a set of three drums—*quinto*, *segundo*, and *tumba*—which function the same as the *requinto* and *seguidoras* of the *bomba*. The ensemble for *yambú* is the same, except that the *segundo* is optional. The *segundo* and *tumba*, when used together, provide the supporting rhythmic structure through interlocking patterns. *Cáscara* and *claves* are used in all three *rumba* forms. *Cáscara* are like the *cuá* of the *bomba*, and together with the *claves* serve the same function of providing the time line around which the other instruments are organized.

Guaguancó, *yambú*, and *columbia*, all musical and dance forms, also use solo voice and chorus. Similarities between *yambú* and *guaguancó* exist in their musical form, which may be divided into three basic sections. The first, *la diana*, is a melodic passage sung in vocables by one of the lead singers or the chorus and serves to cue both the beginning of the song and sectional changes. *El canto* consists of verses sung by a lead singer and stanzas sung by the chorus. The verses may be traditional, improvised, or a combination. The verses of the *canto* thus provide a framework within which the singer can display his poetic and improvisational ability in addition to his knowledge of the traditional repertoire. The verses may also be traded off between two lead singers who enter into a sung verbal duel to see who can be more creative in his use of humor, irony, and metaphor. The final section of the piece, called *rumba* or *el montuno*, switches to a call and response between lead singer and chorus. Although lead singers may take turns initiating the calls, the element of verbal competition that characterizes the *canto* section is not present.

The main distinction between *yambú* and *guaguancó*—other than that *yambú* is slower—is the dance that occurs in the *montuno* section of each. In *guaguancó* the dance is a competition between male and female in which the man attempts to symbolically conquer the woman by the execution of a pelvic thrust known as *vacunao*. While this competition is taking place, the *quinto* interacts with the dancers by responding to their movements. The element of competition does not exist in the *montuno* section of *yambú*; rather, the couples jointly give an elaborate display of expertise. That the *vacunao* is consciously avoided can be seen in the frequent call of the lead singer: *"En el yambú no se vacuna* [as sung], *caballeros"* ("In the *yambú* there is no *vacunao*, gentlemen").

Columbia differs from *yambú* and *guaguancó* in several respects. The latter are in duple meter; *columbia* is in triple meter. *Columbia* has no *diana* section; it has an introductory section, sometimes called *llorao,* in which the lead singer calls his chorus to sound their presence. In *columbia* the dance in the *montuno* section is for men only, and the movements allude to personages in the Abakuá secret society as well as display the dancer's virtuosity. Competition exists between the dancer and the *quintador,* who interact closely. The texts of *guaguancó* and *yambú* are almost always in Spanish, but *columbia* texts include many phrases borrowed from and alluding to the African-derived Abakuá or Lucumí.

Son

Son is a synthesis of various African- and Spanish-derived Cuban musical expressions. It gained widespread popularity in Cuba by the 1920s and internationally in the late twenties and early thirties. *Son* evolved from the *changui* in Oriente Province in the 1800s and was brought to Havana at the turn of the century. In Havana *son* became a popular musical expression of working class people in the early 1900s when it became a vehicle for musically presenting and referring to a host of other musical expressions such as the African-derived *rumba, Santería* and *Abakuá* and the Spanish-derived *décima* and *guajira* (nostalgic solo song accompanied by *tres,* a 6- or 9-stringed guitar-like instrument). While these forms continued to flourish in the communities, by the second decade of the 1900s *son* had become the most popular form of musical expression of Cubans at all levels of society. Through its synthesis of African- and Spanish-derived music styles appealing to all Cubans, the *son* became the equivalent of a Cuban national music and presented a range of musical styles to which many people would otherwise have had limited access.

There have been three recognizable stages in the development of *son,* typified by three groups: Sexteto Habanero, Septeto Nacional and the *conjuntos* (small bands) of Arsenio Rodriguez. By 1918 Sexteto Habanero had started to crystallize what was to become the typical *son conjunto* sound: three voices, string bass, *tres, maracas, bongos, claves,* trumpet and guitar. In the late 1920s Septeto Nacional began to expand on the *son* style established by Habanero. Nacional's sound was characterized by tighter vocal harmonies, expanded melodic range, less freedom for rhythmic improvisation, less rhythmic complexity and a faster tempo.

In the 1930s *son* also became popular in Puerto Rico when musicians there adopted the *son* style into their repertoire. The popularity of *son* continued with the migrations of Cubans and Puerto Ricans to New York.

In the late 1930s Arsenio Rodríguez expanded the *son* sound to incorporate many of the African-derived elements that had been simplified or merely referred to by the earlier *son conjuntos.* Most notably he adapted the form and rhythmic structure of *guaguancó* to *son conjunto* style. Arsenio was able to achieve a synthesis of African- and Spanish-derived elements while maintaining the integrity of both. His innovations included addition of a cowbell, conga drum, second and third trumpet and piano; incorporation of the *tumbao,* a repeated rhythmic pattern resulting from interlocking rhythms played by bass and conga; integration of the rhythm section so as to achieve a melodic-rhythmic unity based on *clave;* expansion of the role of *tres* as a solo instrument; introduction of a *montuno* section—also called *mambo*—for melodic solos with rhythmic back-up; and expansion of song texts to include philosophical statements of Arsenio's sentiments about Cuba, community life and ethnic pride. Arsenio's *sones* came to be called *son montunos.* It was the *montuno*—or *mambo*—section that was the basis for the mambo craze that started in the 1940s and that strongly influenced Latin popular music in New York. Since the 1960s, *son* has included more elements of *rúmba* than ever before.

Salsa

Salsa is to Latinos as Soul is to blacks. The word connotes a feeling as well as a variety of musical traditions that have been redefined and reinterpreted in the context of the Latin popular music scene in New York. Cuban music provides the basis for salsa, but as early as the thirties the Cuban forms had become popular in Puerto Rico. By that time in New York a sizable Latin community had begun to develop, which was tuned in to the Cuban styles and which had been hearing them in the uptown dance halls and nightclubs. Machito, a Cuban who was performing with one of the uptown bands, formed his own group—Machito and His Afro-Cubans—around 1940. The group included Mario Bauza, who had years of experience as a jazz trumpeter with numerous black swing bands. Bauza expanded the size and role of the Latin horn section, using compositional concepts of the black jazz bands, and integrated it with the full Afro-Cuban rhythm section. Thus Machito's group set the stage for a growing relationship between jazz and Latin music that led to the creation of a distinctly New York Latin sound.

In the late forties two highly influential Puerto Rican big-band leaders emerged. Tito Puente and Tito Rodriguez, together with Machito, elaborated on the mambo form and set off the mambo craze of the fifties. Somewhat later a second fad hit New York. *Cha-cha-cha* was brought to New York by Cuban *charanga* orchestras, which consisted of several violins and one flute backed by a rhythm section. *Cha-cha-cha* was also incorporated into the Latin big bands. The mambo and the cha-cha reached a tremendous non-Latino audience and created a dance fad that lasted throughout the fifties.

In addition to the bands that consisted largely of New York Puerto Ricans, popular Cuban artists came to New York to perform. They brought their charts with them and hired the New York musicians to back them up, thus expanding the training ground for young New York Puerto Rican musicians. This training was the foundation of what came to be known in the late sixties as *salsa*.

Until the cessation of diplomatic relations with Cuba in 1962, the interaction between the New York and Cuban music scenes formed the basis for parallel musical development. After 1962 the Cuban musical forms as adopted by Puerto Ricans began to move in directions that further defined the music as a distinctly New York phenomenon. Two general tendencies can be discerned. The first reflects the contact between the Puerto Rican and black communities in New York. By the late sixties there was a large population of bilingual second-generation New York Puerto Ricans whose ties were to both the island and New York. Interaction between blacks and Puerto Ricans was facilitated by overlapping community boundaries and by participation in many of the same educational and recreational institutions. The strength, success and cultural manifestations of the movement for black identity had an important impact on young Puerto Ricans. As one musical result of this interaction, boogaloo, a black musical and dance form that gained tremendous popularity in the mid-sixties was adapted by Puerto Rican musicians and reinterpreted as Latin *bugalú*. It used standard *salsa* instrumentation (horns, piano, bass, congas, *timbales*, bongos, *campana*, and *güiro*) plus trap drums. The rhythmic structure was altered to accent the second and fourth beats (the backbeats), a characteristic feature of black music, and the lyrics were sung in both Spanish and English.

Latin *bugalú* was an attempt to break away from the strict Latin audience and to expand into the mass entertainment industry. But the relationships between Latin and black music were not solely economically motivated. To Puerto Rican musicians who had grown up listening to both Latin and black popular music, the latter offered a logical source for new musical ideas.

The second tendency was to look to the traditional musics of the various Hispanic peoples living in New York. Before 1965 popular Latin music in New York was based primarily on Cuban forms. A notable exception was Rafael Cortijo and his vocalist Ismael Rivera, who as early as 1957 introduced *bomba* and *plena* into the *conjunto* format. The Dominican *merengue* gained solid popularity in the fifties, but it was not adapted to *conjunto* instrumentation until the sixties. At this time, forms such as the Colombian *cumbia* and Puerto Rican *jíbaro* music were also being interpreted and presented in a popular-music idiom under the rubric of salsa. Thus *salsa* today is a vehicle for the expression of many musical forms associated with different Hispanic people coexisting in New York.

Roberta Singer and Robert Friedman both hold Ph.D.'s in Folklore and Ethnomusicology from Indiana University. Dr. Singer is currently the Director of Music Programs at City Lore: The New York Center for Urban Folk Culture. Dr. Friedman is currently completing work on a graduate degree in Social Work at Columbia University.

Further Readings:

Bergman, Billy. *Hot Sauces: Latin and Caribbean Pop* (New York: Quill Books, 1985).

Gonzalez-Wippler, Migene. *Santeria: African Magic in Latin America* (NY: The Julian Press, 1973).

Mintz, Sidney, and Sally Price. *Caribbean Contours* (Baltimore: John Hopkins University Press, 1985).

Roberts, John Storm. *The Latin Tinge* (Tivoli: Original Music, 1979).

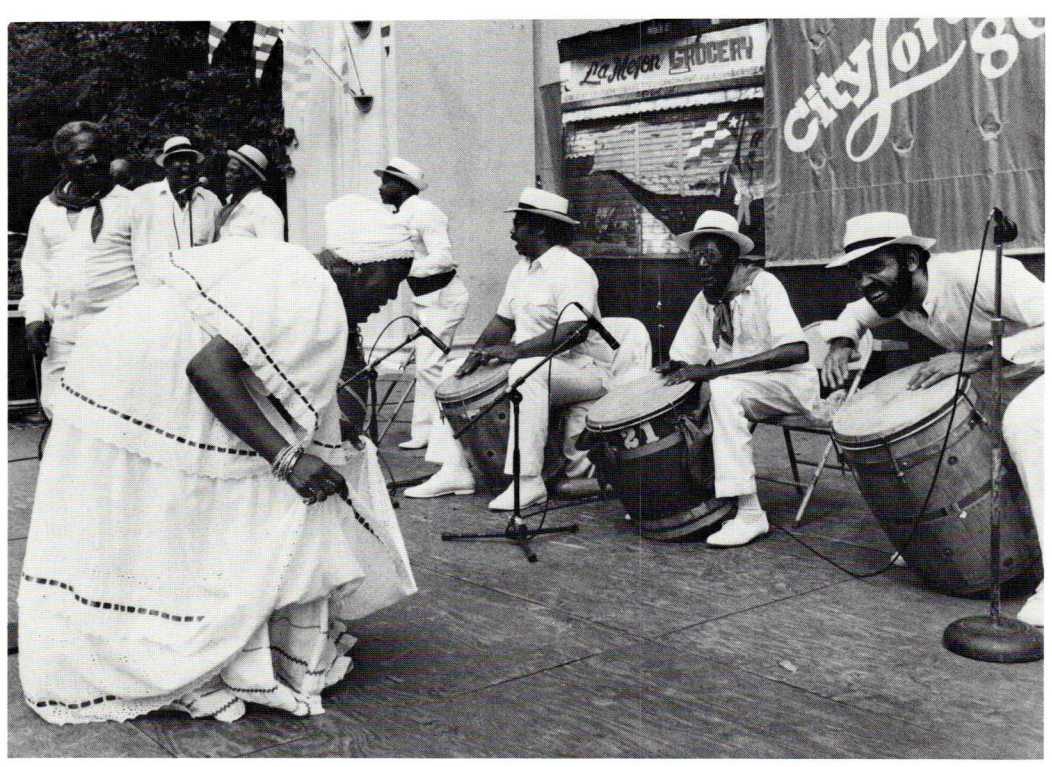

Los Pleneros de la 21 performing a Puerto Rican *Bomba*.

Cajun Music: A Louisiana French Tradition
by Barry Jean Ancelet

Cajun music is a Louisiana hybrid, a blend of cultural influences with an identity which accordion maker and musician Marc Savoy of Eunice describes in culinary terms: "It's a blend of ingredients, like a gumbo in which different spices and flavors combine to make a new taste." Indeed, like Cajun cooking and culture in general, Cajun music blends elements of American Indian, Scots-Irish, Spanish, German, Anglo-American and Afro-Caribbean musics with a rich stock of western French folk traditions.

Most of Louisiana's French population descends from the Acadians, the French colonists who began settling at Port Royal, Acadia in 1604. They remained outside mainstream communication between France and its larger, more important colony, New France, though their isolation was frequently disturbed by the power struggle between the English and French colonial empires. Acadia changed hands back and forth until the Treaty of Utrecht in 1713, when England gained permanent possession of the colony and renamed it Nova Scotia. The Acadians were eventually deported from their homeland in 1755 by local British authorities after years of political and religious tension. In 1765, after 10 years of wandering, many Acadians began to arrive in Louisiana, determined to recreate their society. Within a generation these exiles had so firmly reestablished themselves as a people that they became the dominant culture in South Louisiana, absorbing other ethnic groups around them. Most of the French Creoles (descendants of earlier French settlers), Spanish, Germans, and Anglo-Americans in the region eventually adopted the traditions and language of this new society, thus creating the South Louisiana mainstream. The Acadians, in turn, borrowed many traits from these other cultures, and this cross-cultural exchange produced a new Louisiana-based community—the Cajuns.

The Acadians' contact with these various cultures contributed to the development of new musical styles and repertoire. From Indians, they learned wailing singing styles and new dance rhythms; from Blacks, they learned the blues, percussion techniques, and improvisational singing; from Anglo-Americans, they learned new fiddle tunes to accompany Virginia reels, square dances and hoedowns. The Spanish contributed the guitar and even a few tunes. Refugees and their slaves who arrived from Saint-Domingue at the turn of the nineteenth century brought with them a syncopated West Indian beat. Jewish-German immigrants began importing diatonic accordions (invented in Vienna in 1828) toward the end of the nineteenth century when Acadians and Black Creoles began to show an interest in the instruments. They blended these elements to create a new music just as they were synthesizing the same cultures to create Cajun society.

The turn of the twentieth century was a formative period in the development of Louisiana French music. Some of its most influential musicians were the Black Creoles who brought a strong, rural blues element into Cajun music. Simultaneously Blacks influenced the parallel development of zydeco music, later refined by Clifton Chenier. Although fiddlers such as Dennis McGee and Sady Courville still composed tunes, the accordion was rapidly becoming the mainstay of traditional dance bands. Limited in the number of notes and keys it could play in, it simplified Cajun music; songs which could not be played on the accordion faded from the active repertoire. Meanwhile, fiddlers were often relegated to playing a duet accompaniment or a simple percussive second line below the accordion's melodic lead.

By the mid-1930s, Cajuns were reluctantly, though inevitably, becoming Americanized. Their French language was banned from schools throughout South Louisiana as America, caught in the "melting pot" ideology, tried to homogenize its diverse ethnic and cultural elements. In South Louisiana, speaking French was not only against the rules, it became increasingly unpopular as Cajuns attempted to escape the stigma attached to their culture. New highways and improved transportation opened this previously isolated area to the rest of the country, and the Cajuns began to imitate their Anglo-American neighbors in earnest.

The social and cultural changes of the 1930s and 1940s were clearly reflected in the music recorded in this period. The slick programming on radio (and later on television) inadvertently forced the comparatively unpolished traditional sounds underground. The accordion faded from the scene, partly because the old-style music had lost popularity and partly because the instruments were unavailable from Germany during the war. As western swing and bluegrass sounds from Texas and Tennessee swept the country, string bands which imitated the music of Bob Wills and the Texas Playboys and copied Bill Monroe's "high lonesome sound" sprouted across South Louisiana. Freed from the limitations imposed by the accordion, string bands readily absorbed various outside influences. Dancers across South Louisiana were shocked in the mid-1930s to hear music which came not only from the bandstand, but also from the opposite end of the dance hall through speakers powered by a Model-T behind the building. The electric steel guitar was added to the standard instrumentation and drums replaced the triangle as Cajuns continued to experiment with new sounds borrowed from their Anglo-American neighbors. As amplification made it unnecessary for fiddlers to bear down with the bow to be audible, they developed a lighter, lilting touch, moving away from the soulful styles of earlier days.

By the late 1940s, the music recorded by commercial producers signalled an unmistakable tendency toward Americanization. Yet an undercurrent of traditional music persisted. It resurfaced with the music of Iry Lejeune, who accompanied the Oklahoma Tornadoes in 1948 to record *La Valse du Pont d'Amour* in the turn-of-the-century Louisiana style and in French. The recording was an unexpected success, presaging a revival of the earlier style, and Iry Lejeune became a pivotal figure in a Cajun music revival. Dance halls providing traditional music flourished, and musicians such as Lawrence Walker, Austin Pitre and Nathan Abshire brought their accordions out of the closet and once again performed old-style Cajun music, while local companies began recording them. Cajun music, though bearing the marks of Americanization, was making a dramatic comeback, just as interest in the culture and language quickened before the 1955 bicentennial celebration of the Acadian exile.

Alan Lomax, a member of the Newport Folk Festival Foundation who had become interested in Louisiana French folk music during a field trip with his father in the 1930s, encouraged the documentation and preservation of Cajun music. In the late 1950s, Harry Oster began recording a musical spectrum of Cajun music which ranged from unaccompanied ballads to contemporary dance tunes. His collection, which stressed the evolution of the music, attracted the attention of local activists, such as Paul Tate and Revon Reed. The work of Oster and Lomax was noticed by the Newport Foundation, which sent fieldworkers Ralph Rinzler and Mike Seeger to South Louisiana. Cajun dance bands had played at the National Folk Festival as early as 1935, but little echo of these performances reached Louisiana. Rinzler and Seeger, seeking the unadorned roots of Cajun music, chose Gladius Thibodeaux, Louis "Vinesse" Lejeune and Dewey Balfa to represent Louisiana at the 1964 Newport Folk Festival. Their "gutsy," unamplified folk music made the Louisiana cultural establishment uneasy, for such "unrefined" sounds embarrassed the upwardly mobile Cajuns who considered the music chosen for the Newport festival crude—"nothing but chanky-chank."

The instincts of the Newport festival organizers proved well-founded, as huge crowds gave the old-time music standing ovations. Dewey Balfa was so moved that he returned to Louisiana determined to bring the message home. He began working on a small scale among his friends and family in Mamou, Basile and Eunice. The Newport Folk Foundation, under the guidance of Lomax, provided money and fieldworkers to the new Louisiana Folk Foundation "to water the roots." With financial support and outside approval, local activists became involved in preserving the music, language and culture. Traditional music contests and concerts were organized at events such as the Abbeville Dairy Festival, the Opelousas Yambilee and the Crowley Rice Festival.

In 1968, the state of Louisiana officially recognized the Cajun cultural revival which had been brewing under the leadership of the music community and political leaders, such as Dudley LeBlanc and Roy Theriot. In that year, it created the Council for the Development of French in Louisiana (CODOFIL) which, under the chairmanship of James Domengeaux, began its efforts on

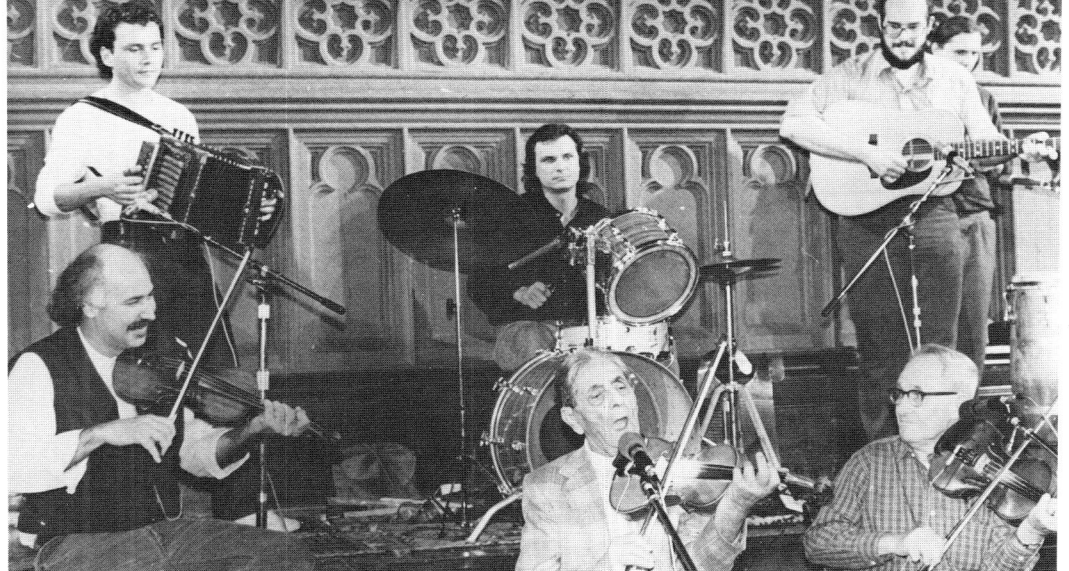
Beausoleil with Dennis McGee and Sady Courville.

political, psychological and educational fronts to erase the stigma Louisianans had long attached to the French language and culture. The creation of French classes in elementary schools dramatically reversed the policy which had formerly barred the language from the schoolgrounds.

Domengeaux's efforts were not limited to the classroom. Influenced by Rinzler and Balfa, CODOFIL organized a first *Tribute to Cajun Music* festival in 1974 with a concert designed to present an historical overview of Cajun music from its origins to modern styles. The echo had finally come home. Dewey Balfa's message of cultural self-esteem was enthusiastically received by an audience of over 12,000.

Because of its success, the festival became an annual celebration of Cajun music and culture. It not only provided exposure for the musicians but presented them as cultural heroes. Young performers were attracted to the revalidated Cajun music scene, while local French movement officials, realizing the impact of the grass-roots, began to stress the native Louisiana French culture. Balfa's dogged pursuit of cultural recognition carried him farther than he had ever expected. In 1977, he received a Folk Artists in the Schools grant from the National Endowment for the Arts to bring his message into elementary school classrooms. Young Cajuns, discovering local models besides country and rock stars, began to perform the music of their heritage. Yet, they did not reject modern sounds totally. Performers such as Michael Doucet and Beausoleil are gradually making their presence known in Cajun music, replacing older musicians on the regular weekend dance hall circuit and representing traditional Cajun music at local and national festivals.

Cajun music seems likely to live for some time to come. The renewed creativity within the tradition, as opposed to slavish imitation of older styles, makes predictions of its disappearance seem hasty. Purists who would resist new instrumentation and styles ignore the fact that change and innovation have always characterized Cajun music— the introduction of the accordion in the late nineteenth century, for instance, or the adding of other instruments in the 1950s, and the influence of the blues, swing, and rock. As Dewey Balfa points out, "When things stop changing, they die. The culture and the music have to breathe and grow, but they have to stay within certain guidelines to be true. And those guidelines are pureness and sincerity." The blending and cultural fusion at the heart of the development of Cajun culture continue to be essential to its music.

Since 1977, Barry Jean Ancelet has been folklorist with the Center for Louisiana Studies of the University of Southwestern Louisiana in Lafayette.

Further Readings:

Ancelet, Barry Jean. *The Makers of Cajun Music* (Austin: University of Texas Press, 1984).

Broven, John. *South to Louisiana: The Music of the Cajun Bayous* (Gretna, LA: Pelican Publishing Company, 1983).

Ruston, William Faulkner. *The Cajuns: From Acadia to Louisiana* (New York: Farrar Straus Giroux, 1979).

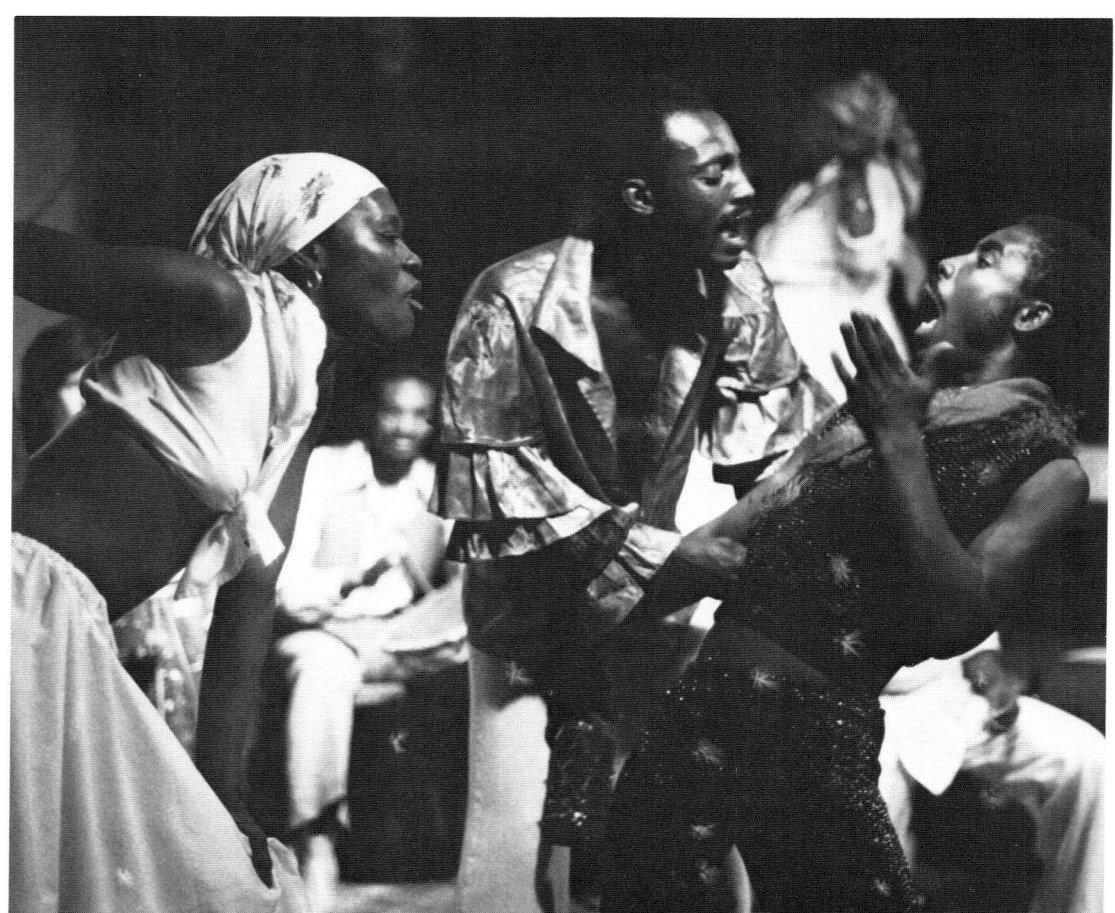

La Troupe Makandal performing a Haitian Voudon Ceremony.

Taking Spirit Time: Vodoun Sounds of Haiti
by Frisner Augustin and Lois Wilcken

The music of Haitian Vodoun begins in the religious system, a syncretic faith comprising beliefs and practices of the descendants of Africans, American Indians, and Roman Catholic Europeans. Scholar Maya Deren argues that certain spirit groups are essentially of Native American (Arawak or Carib) origin. But Vodoun was shaped primarily by Africans brought to Haiti from Togo, Benin, Nigeria, Northwest Africa, Sierra Leone, the Congo Basin, and Angola during the transatlantic slave trade. In 1791, after a long process of coalescence, these various nations united to overthrow the French colonists. Political solidarity resulted in some degree of spiritual solidarity, and today, Vodounists pay homage to nearly two dozen ancestral nations. Added to this fusion of African belief systems is a veneer of Christianity.

The concept of nations is important because it shapes ritual. Haitians remember that it was the spirits of these nations who protected them during slavery and the revolution. They continue to seek the spirits' protection now. During a Vodoun dance, the most dramatic ritual and the one in which music plays its most prominent role, the nations most important to the society holding the dance are saluted in turn. In much of Haiti, the Fon of Dahomey seem to have made the strongest impression on the religion—the word "Vodoun" is a Fon term for spirit, or deity—and so the Fon spirits, known in Haiti as the Rada nation, are saluted first in many dances. In dances held in Port-au-Prince, most of central Haiti, and New York City, the Rada spirits are given the greatest portion of the event, and they are customarily followed in order of salutation by the Djouba, Nago, Pétro, Ibo, Congo, and Gedé nations.

To put their beliefs into action, Vodounists organize themselves into societies. The head of a society is either a *ougan* (priest) or a *manbo* (priestess). His/her principal assistants are the *laplas*, a master of ceremonies; the *ounjenikon*, a song specialist; and the *ounsi*, initiates responsible for a wide range of tasks, such as preparing food for the spirits, pouring libations, carrying the society's flags, wiping the faces of perspiring drummers, and, most important, singing and dancing. Drummers are essential personnel, but they are not necessarily initiates. Finally, there are the *loa*. Loa is a Congolese word that is used today to refer to the most outstanding ancestral spirits. Through a phenomenon called possession in industrial societies, and "getting a spirit" in Haiti, the spirit that animates a living being is temporarily displaced by a loa, who then takes an active role in the dance, often dispensing advice, often sharing the foods that have been prepared for him/her. When the loa departs, the spirit of the living enters the body again.

Just as the organization of the dance is determined by nations, so is the organization of the symbolic systems that articulate it. Music is one of these systems, along with dance, color, food, drink, clothing, and, of course, language. Vodounists identify song, rhythm, and instrumentation as the salient elements of their music, and they classify the items within each by nation. A Vodoun dance opens with songs for the Rada spirits. These loa originated in the courtly, urbanized kingdom of Dahomey. Social hierarchy is observed strictly in their rites, and it is reflected in song. A manbo, oungan, or ounjenikon sings several phrases, and he/she is answered by the chorus of ounsi in the call-and-response style typical of West Africa. The song ends in the solo-chorus alternation of the last line. A dance closes with songs for the Pétro and Gedé nations. The celebrants of these loa, particularly the Pétro, were identified as Creolo (not born in Africa). The fiery, revolutionary character of the Pétros and the overt sexuality of the Gedés show a tendency to dissolve social hierarchy. Correspondingly, the performance of these songs is more democratic than the performance of Rada songs. Anyone may initiate a song, and sometimes there is heated discussion over what should be sung next. Call-and-response patterns become increasingly irregular.

In Vodoun music, instruments are also used symbolically. Each major nation of loa has its characteristic ensemble, although the Nagos tend to use the Rada set, and the Gedés share with the Pétros. The Rada ensemble comprises three drums and one metal percussion piece. The largest and lowest pitched of the drums is the *maman*, on which the master drummer plays the most skillful and elaborate patterns. Interacting with the maman through a vocabulary of somewhat less intricate patterns is the *ségon*, slightly smaller and higher pitched than the maman. The smallest, highest pitched drum is the *boula*, whose function is to provide a steady staccato. The metal piece is called *ogan*. It may be a bell, a hoe blade, or anything made of metal. It is struck preferably with a metal stick, and it functions as timekeeper. Finally, the *ason* is a gourd rattle covered with a mesh of snake vertebrae or colored beads; a small bell with clapper is affixed to its handle. The ason is shaken by the oungan/manbo, whose role it is to direct the flow of the dance. It is used only in Rada rites.

The various sets used in Vodoun differ in shape, with some conical and others cylindrical; in tuning system, with some using pegs around the head and others using cords stretched along the body; and in drum head material, with some using cow skin and others goat. There are differences in performance practice, too. Rada drums are struck with sticks, Pétro drums with bare hands. This reflects again the social distinction made between these nations. Pétros are more informal, and drummers feel that playing with hands is less strenuous than playing with sticks. Perhaps the most striking expression of nationhood through performance practice is seen in drumming for the Djouba loa. The master drummer lays his instrument parallel to the ground and sits on it, playing with both hands and feet. Djoubas are spirits of the earth; the drum is lowered to the earth in recognition of their domain.

Rhythm is the hallmark of Vodoun music. Webs of the highest complexity are woven by the interaction of three or more instruments as they maintain a steady pulse together while simultaneously creating patterns that depart from the pulse. Rhythm is also the element that marks the finest symbolic distinctions among the loa. Each nation has its own set of percussion patterns, and often the rhythm and the dance it accompanies are named after their corresponding nation. Nago, for example, is played for the Nago nation, the rhythm Congo for the Congo nation, and so on. However, Yanvalou, a Fon term for praise, is played for the Rada loa. Groupings of nations and divisions among them are reflected in percussion patterns. The basic timekeeping instruments, those that embellish least, show interrelationships among nations, while the master and second drums show distinctions. For example, the ogan and boula parts for Pétro and Banda are the same, while their maman and ségon differ. As noted above, these loa share certain democratic and informal features, yet they are different in temperament and domain.

One of the marks of the master drummer is his ability to execute a *kasé*. This term means "break," and it literally breaks the steady pulse set up by the patterns that precede it. A kasé may stretch time by using a longer pattern; its main points of emphasis may fall in shockingly unexpected places. There is no doubt that the kasé is related to spirit possession. Deren believes that the kasé "empties the head and leaves one without any center around which to stabilize". Under these circumstances, the loa may enter. A master drummer will tell you that he plays a kasé "when I feel the spirit coming."

Drummers consider timbre an essential aspect of rhythm. The color of a drum sound is determined by the way the drum is struck, and Vodoun drummers utilize a palette as broad and varied as that of contemporary Haitian painters. A drum head may be struck at its center, on the rim, or in between with stick or hand. The latter may be flat or cupped, and it may bounce or stop. A portamento (smooth blending of pitch) is achieved by sliding the fingers across the head. And so on. It is vital that these articulations be crisp and distinguishable. They give a pattern a large part of its identity, and drummers have developed a vocabulary for them: bass, tone, *sié* (slide), etc.

There is no vocabulary for duration, but this does not mean that Vodoun drummers fail to consider the temporal aspect of rhythm. The duration that transpires from one sound to the next, as measured in clock time, is insignificant to the Vodoun drummer. What matters to him instead is that his playing is synchronized with an inner pulse, and is somewhat restrained. Self-control is important, and rushing ahead is a major flaw. Most drumming errors are corrected with the admonition "Prann san ou," which literally means "Take your blood." Its figurative meaning, as expressed by Haitians who speak English, is "Take your time." A rhythmic error, then, is not a failure to measure duration as much as it is a failure to relax.

Vodoun music is a dynamic tradition, always alert to the world around it. What began as a musical salute to an association of distinct nations continues to fuse. The differences between Ibo and Congo music, for example, grow progressively more difficult to define. There are fewer drum batteries today than there once were. In recent dances in New York, trumpet and electric flute have joined the chorus of ounsi. Vodoun music has always been, and will continue to be, an evolving body of knowledge that changes and enriches itself along with the people who make it.

Epilogue
On Becoming a Drummer

I must have been fifteen. I go to a Vodoun ceremony, and I watch the way my uncle plays, and all the guys. And I keep watching. I tell the guy who plays the bell, "Can I do something?" I'm scared to tell him that, because this guy is bigger than me. And he says, "Frisner, can you do it?" I say, "Well, let me try." This guy gives me the bell, and I play it. And he doesn't take it away from me; he lets me still play. And I say, "Oh, I'm good!"

After I get tired of the bell, I tell the guy on the boula, "Give me the boula." And people say, "Oh, Frisner, are you drunk? You play bell, you play boula..." I say, "Listen, I do everything one at a time." Right? Then I say, "Let me do the ségon now." The guy says, "Oh, Frisner, you're terrible now! You want to get everything at one time?" I say, "Yeah!"

The guy playing maman is watching me. "Frisner, you want to play maman, too?" I say, "No, not now, but I'm going to get it soon." And as soon as I tell the guy that, Ogoun is coming—you know, the spirit. He's very heavy, Ogoun. But Ogoun is my favorite spirit, and Ogoun is happy to see me play the drum. He tells me, "Frisner, I'm going to get you to play for me." And I tell Ogoun, "You think I play good?" He says, "Yeah. If you don't play good, I'll tell you to get off the drum."

And Ogoun says, "Frisner, I'm going to help you."

Lois Wilcken, a Ph.D. candidate in Columbia University's Ethnomusicology Program, has done extensive field research in Brooklyn's Haitian community. Frisner Augustin, a native of Port of Prince, Haiti, is a master drummer and instructor of percussion at Hunter College.

Further Readings:

Courlander, Harold. *Haiti Singing* (New York: Cooper Square Publishers, Inc., 1973).

Deren, Maya. *Divine horsemen: The Living Gods of Haiti* (New Paltz, NY: McPherson & Co., 1953, 1984).

Metraux, Alfred. *Voodoo in Haiti* (NY: Schocken Books, 1972).

Moreau de St. Mery. *Description topographique, physique, civile, politique, et historique de la partie francaise de l'isle Saint-Domingue.* Blanche Morel et Etienne Taillemite, eds. (Paris: Société de l'Histoire des Colonies Francaise et Librairie Larose, 1958).

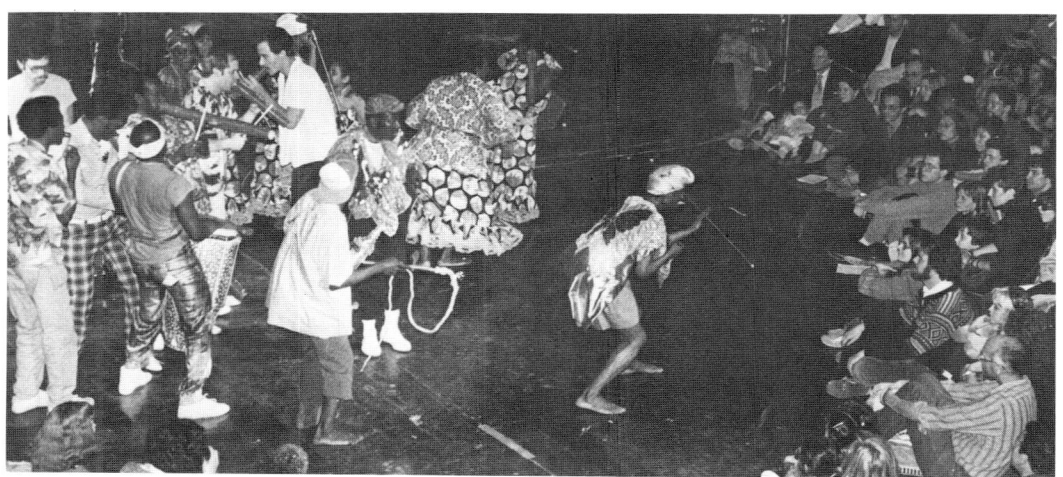

La Troupe Makandal performing a Haitian *Rara*.

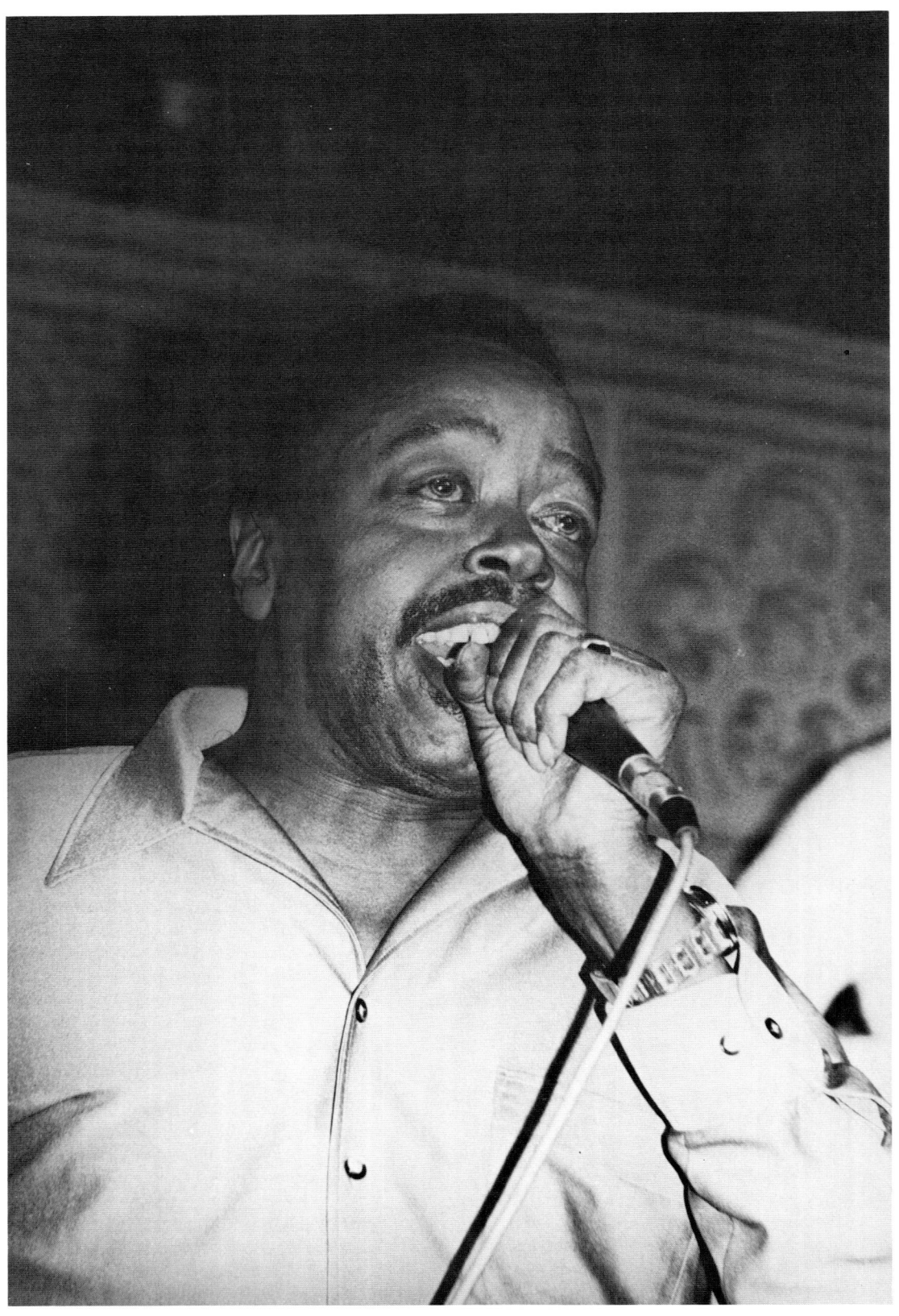

Carey Bell.

Mexican Traditions: The Son Jarocho
by Daniel Sheehy

Regionalism has long played a dominant role in Mexican cultural life. In pre-Columbian times, the Mexican landscape was populated by a myriad of Amerindian groups speaking many different languages. When the Spaniards began arriving in 1519, they brought with them a strong heritage of regional distinctions—Basques, Galicians, Valencians, Andalusians, and many others. The large numbers of African slaves forcibly brought in the sixteenth, seventeenth, and eighteenth centuries to labor in the fields and mines of New Spain (as Mexico was called prior to independence) came from culturally diverse tribal groups in west and central Africa. As colonial times (1521-1810) progressed, the culturally mixed *mestizo* population increased in numbers and in cultural and political importance, ultimately accounting for the great majority of Mexico's inhabitants. Over those three centuries during which the new, uniquely Mexican *mestizo* character of its people took shape, the forces of regionalism—geographic isolation, differences in climate, economy, topography, and ethnic mix, among others—were at work, forging yet newer lines of regional distinctions. By the nineteenth century, mention of many diverse regional traditions of dialect, dress, foodways, celebrations and music were commonplace in the writings of Mexicans and foreign travelers alike.

Despite the glossing over of many regional distinctions in the twentieth century by the loud voice of the centralized popular electronic media, many of the stronger regional musical traditions prevail and some have been assimilated in varying degrees into the popular notion of Mexican national identity. Probably the most well known Mexican popular music with strong folk roots is that of the *mariachi* ensemble. At the turn of this century, the mariachi was an ensemble of string instruments—usually diatonic harp, violin, and local guitars called *guitarra de golpe* (also known as *jarana*) and *vihuela*—limited to the area around the west Mexican state of Jalisco. As the financial rewards and prestige presented by the advent of radio, recording and, later, films attracted rural musicians from the Mexican hinterlands to Mexico City, it also led to changes in traditional musical styles, as they adapted to the tastes and demands of producers and the new, more urban audiences. In the mariachi, trumpets, the more suave-sounding standard guitar, and the *guitarron* bass guitar were added, as the harp and raucous *guitarra de golpe* fell into near disuse. Gradually, the harmonic, rhythmic and melodic idioms of commercial popular music augmented the few traditional dance and song genres of the mariachi and its limited vocabulary of chords and meters.

Farther to the west and north; the *banda* (wind and percussion band) has attained a certain primacy among the *mestizo* population of the states of Sinaloa and Zacatecas. In the nineteenth century, bands composed brass, woodwind and percussion instruments were the vogue throughout Mexico. Many towns built bandstands in the middle of their central plazas, where their citizens would come on weekends and special occasions to socialize and listen to European light classics, traditional Mexican tunes arranged for the banda, and original compositions, usually in old modes such as the waltz, by Mexican composers. Out of this band tradition came the *banda sinaloense* (Sinaloan band) with its trumpets, clarinets, valve trombones, sousaphone bass, and stationary bass drum with cymbal and snare drum. In neighboring Zacatecas, the *tamborazo zacatecano* evolved, much like the banda sinaloense but with saxophones instead of clarinets and the bass drum, cymbals, and snare drums of the typical marching band.

In Chiapas and Oaxaca in southern Mexico, the wooden marimba became the best known local traditional musical ensemble. Of African origin in structure, the marimba is found throughout Central America and in a slightly different form in Colombia. Today, the marimba is found all over Mexico, performed either alone or together with a few other instruments such as bass and snare drum, *güiro* (rasp), and string bass.

To the north, the mix of longstanding Mexican inhabitants and the mid-19th century influx of immigrants from Central Europe led to the creation of yet another regional music, called *música norteña* in Mexico and *conjunto* or *música tejana* on the American side of the border in Texas. The key musical instrument in *música norteña* is the button accordion, played in a style unique to the region. It is most often accompanied by a three-string upright bass called *tololoche* and a large guitar with

12 strings called *bajo sexto*, though on the American side of the border, an electric bass and drum trap set are most often used instead of the string bass.

On the east coast of Mexico in the state of Veracruz is found the style of folk music known as *música jarocha*. The *jarochos*, as *Veracruzanos* are often called, are thought by many to possess traditions of music, dance and dress more similar to those of southern Spain than are found in any other part of Mexico. This may indeed be the case, particularly in view of the fact that until this century, the port city of Veracruz was the main gateway to Spain and the outside world. At the same time, however, some of the heaviest concentrations of African immigrants were in Veracruz, and these ancestors of present-day *jarochos* undoubtedly left their mark in the course of the development of *música jarocha*.

The music of the *jarochos* is animated, witty, picaresque, and spiced with a heavy dose of spontaneous improvisation, both in instrumental performance and in the creation of song texts. The instruments of the region are clearly of Spanish derivation, but are nevertheless unlike any other. The three main *jarocho* instruments found today are the *arpa*, a 32-to-36-string harp standing about five feet tall; the *jarana*, a small, eight-string (with three double courses) guitar that provides the rhythmic and harmonic framework for the music; and the *requinto*, a melody-playing, four-string guitar plucked with a four-inch pick fashioned of cow horn or a plastic comb. Singing is most often done in alternation. Singers may trade off in singing short verses or a lead singer (*pregonero*, or "caller") may sing the first portion of a phrase and one or more of the remaining musicians will either repeat or answer that portion. Tempos are almost always fast-moving.

Virtually all the pieces in the traditional repertory of *jarocho* musicians are called *sones*. The musical genre known as *son* evolved during the Mexican colonial period and became the most widespread and popular musical expression of the mestizo population. Through time, *sones* were shaped by regional tastes and circumstances and further evolved into regionally demarcated types of *son*, each with a distinctive accompanying instrumentation, rhythmic and melodic preferences, and repertory. In Veracruz, the total repertory of traditional regional *sones* is thought not to exceed 70 in number. In addition, a few *sones* composed in the 1920s and 1930s, though somewhat different in structure and style, have crept into the repertories of traditional musicians. One example of this is "Tilingo Lingo," composed by Lino Carrillo.

Most traditional *jarocho* musicians come from the ranchlands and fishing ports of Veracruz. Many continue to work as small ranchers or fishermen, traveling to tourist centers in slow times to augment their incomes. In and around Veracruz, Mandinga, Boca del Rio, Alvarado, and other coastal towns, they perform in the many outdoor seafood restaurants that cater mainly to Mexican tourists and local Veracruzanos. A few are occasionally hired to accompany *ballet folkloricos* recreating the sights and sounds of the now rare traditional social occasion for the *son jarocho*, the *fandango*. Prior to the 1940s, fandangos, community celebrations with *musica jarocha* and dancing prominent, were peak social events in rural Veracruz.

Since the beginning in the 1930s of the large-scale migrations of regional folk musicians to Mexico City, many *jarocho* musicians with aspirations of professional musical careers have migrated there and to other cities in Mexico and the southwest United States in search of paid performing and recording opportunities. Through this migration and the spread of *musica jarocha* through the commercial electronic media, *musica jarocha* has become widely known both as a symbol of regional identity and as an important living part of Mexico's national patrimony.

Dan Sheehy holds a Ph.D. in Ethnomusicology from UCLA, where he specialized in Mexican Mestizo music.

Music of the Peruvian Highlands

by Thomas Turino

The richness of contemporary Andean musical traditions must be viewed in terms of great regional and ethnic/class diversity, as well as with regard to the different ways in which the European and indigenous cultures have interacted since the Spanish conquest in 1532. With regard to the performance of highland musical instruments and genres, three basic types of manifestations may be identified. First, there is a distinct indigenous musical-aesthetic system within certain Indian communities in Ecuador, Peru and Bolivia. While European influence has penetrated even the most isolated highland areas, in the indigenous context Western innovations are largely incorporated and redefined according to Andean patterns, and a continuity of indigenous elements remains dominant.

Secondly, there is a distinct musical culture among highland *mestizos* (mixed Andean and Western cultural heritage) in which European and Andean elements and aesthetics have been integrally fused over a period of centuries. Since the 1960s a third musical movement has emerged. This urban-revivalist style, which is the best known internationally, evolved in cities in the Andean area largely among middle-class youth and university students. In contrast to the indigenous situation where occidental innovations (e.g., stringed instruments) are incorporated into the Andean system, the latter represents the inverse, with Andean forms (instruments and genres) being reinterpreted largely according to urban-occidental aesthetic values and patterns. These three types of Andean music in Peru will be contrasted briefly below with regard to form, aesthetic values and performance contexts after an introduction to some musical instruments of the area.

Instruments

Pre-Columbian Andean musical instruments have been well documented by archeologists and in historical records written close to the time of the Spanish conquest (see Stevenson 1968). These include winds, drums, and percussion instruments. Among the winds, single and double row panpipes, *antara*s (known generically today as *zampoña*s in Spanish and *siku*s in Aymara) were used in the highlands and among pre-Inca coastal cultures. They were made of ceramic, cane or bone, and their size, the number of tubes, and their scales varied widely. Studies regarding these instruments cast doubt on the predominance of pentatonicism for the pre-Columbian period (Stevenson 1968; Haeberli 1979). There is evidence that double-row panpipes were played in "interlocking fashion," as will be described below, as well as single-row instruments in ensembles with different octaves, and possibly harmonic voicing (Garcilaso 1960:94; Rossel 1977; Valencia 1982). The pre-Columbian practice of accompanying winds with drums, maintained today, is also documented in the archeological record.

Clay, metal, and conch-shell trumpets (without stops) were also widely used in Inca and pre-Inca musical cultures. Vertical end-notched flutes, such as the contemporary *kena* (quena), were also used, made out of bone, clay or cane. Again the number of stops and scales vary for these instruments. In pre-Hispanic times vertical end-notched flutes were known as *pinkullu* (*pingollo*, etc.; see Guaman Poma 1980). Side-blown flutes have also been documented for pre-Columbian coastal culture (Stevenson 1968). A small double-headed drum known then and now as *tinya* was used; as were larger drums.

After the Spanish conquest, stringed instruments such as the diatonic harp and violin, as well as guitars, *vihuela*s, *laud*s, and *bandurria*-type instruments were introduced. The harp-violin combination was widely diffused among indigenous people by Catholic missionaries early in the colonial period, and these traditions are still important in Peru and Ecuador. The Andean *charango*, usually a small guitar-shaped instrument with a flat or round back (made of wood or sometimes armadillo shell), and between four and fifteen strings (divided into four or five courses) came into being around 1700. This instrument, a product of European and Andean culture contact, was first used by mestizos and was also adopted by the indigenous population.

The existence of pre-Columbian vertical duct-flutes, with a "whistle-like" mouthpiece, is not clearly documented in the archeological or historical record. Hence, the large variety of contemporary duct flutes played by the indigenous population known presently as *pinkullu*s or *pinkillu*s, *tarka*s, *roncadore*s, etc., seems to be a post-conquest innovation. In this century, the accordion and other European instruments such as the saxophone and clarinet have become important highland traditions in certain parts of Peru, as has the brass band tradition throughout the sierra.

Indigenous Musical Culture

While there is great regional variety in indigenous music in highland Peru, certain aesthetic and contextual features unify it as a distinct and coherent system. In terms of aesthetic principles the following generalizations hold for most regional traditions. First, there is a preference for high pitch, and a thick or "fat" sound. Both features may be perceived in the strident, nasal Andean vocal style (in which young women are the preferred singers), as well as in most flute traditions in which over-blowing techniques are consistently used and the lower octave rarely heard. End-notched, duct, side-blown flutes, and panpipes are blown in such a way as to create an airy sound (air spills over the mouthpiece) and, with the exception of panpipes, abundant overtones, resulting in a "thick" sound. The multiple thin metal strings and strumming style preferred by Indian charango players, in contrast with the mestizo plucked style on nylon strings, also produces a "fat" sound. The instrument's small size aids in attaining higher-pitched tunings. Vibrato is absent from indigenous vocal, wind, and string performance.

Indigenous Andean music is also characterized by a high degree of external and internal repetition. That is, a single short piece, perhaps lasting a minute, will be performed for as many as twenty or more repetitions. The structure of most indigenous Andean genres includes two or three repeated sections (AA, BB, CC) and there is often a high degree of internal repetition of musical motives between the sections.

For the most part, different types of melody instruments are not mixed in indigenous musical culture. Thus panpipes are only played in ensemble with panpipes, pinkillus with other pinkillus, etc. In Cusco the indigenous charango tradition follows this pattern, and charangos are performed only with other charangos to accompany vocals and dancing.

In the indigenous context, musical/dance performance tends to be a non-specialist, communal affair in keeping with the collective nature of indigenous society. The Aymara panpipe, *pinkillu* (cane duct flute, 5 or 6 holes), *tarka* (wooden 6-hole duct flute) and end-notched flute (e.g., *pulipuli*s and *choquela*s) traditions in the state of Puno—where any male community member is welcome to join the ensemble—represent the best examples of this. These different indigenous wind instruments tend to be played in large ensembles (10-50 players, males only) accompanied by drums. So too, in certain communities in southern Cusco, all young Quechua males perform charango as non-specialists as part of the courting process (Turinio 1983).

The "hocket" technique for the double-row panpipe, used consistently in the indigenous context, is also an obvious manifestation of the communal/reciprocal nature of indigenous musical performance. The two rows of the panpipe (a diatonic scale alternates between them) are divided between a pair of musicians, each one supplying the notes of the melody contained on his row in interlocking fashion. In Puno, solo performance is minimal, and the value of "playing as one," or group blend, in which no individual player stands out, is stressed in most instrumental traditions.

Indigenous musical/dance genres are most often identified by the specific contexts in which they are used. The music is predominantly in duple meter with a syncopated rhythm, but the melodic shape and scales (between 3 and 7 pitches) vary according to region, context, and instrumental tradition. The instruments themselves are also strictly linked to specific contexts. Thus, in the state of Junin the *wakrapuku* (also called *cacho*, a circular cow horn trumpet) is used for the Fiesta of Santiago, and at other times of the year, for the ritual marking of animals. The different pieces performed would be labelled with regard to their function in the ceremony ("entrance", "marking music", etc.), and the genre as a whole is called *marcación del ganado* (marking the herds). In Puno, for example, tarkas are only used during Carnaval, and the dance genre performed is called *Carnavales*. Pinkillus are performed for agricultural rituals and community dancing during the Carnaval season, and for the ancestors in *Todos los Santos* (November 2). Panpipes in Puno are performed for dancing at fiestas in the months of April-October, or for weddings at any time of year, and charangos in southern Cusco are used for courting and for potato planting music (*papa tarpuy*). While in the indigenous context fiesta names are often derived from Catholic or European tradition—"Carnival", "Fiesta of the Cross," etc.—the content of such fiestas most often relates to the indigenous religion, agricultural cycle, political system, work and life cycles.

Mestizo Musical Culture

While in certain areas in Peru, the charango, the harp, and the violin have been incorporated into the indigenous musical culture, string music is largely the domain of *mestizo* musicians. Ensembles composed of guitars, mandolins, violins, harp, charango, vocals, and sometimes accordion and/or harmonica and kena are a mainstay of mestizo music throughout the Peruvian sierra. In addition, Western brass band instrumentation (derived from the military band tradition) is very important for mestizo dance and fiesta occasions, as is the *orquesta* of Junin composed of saxophones, clarinets, harp and violin. The mixing of classes of melodic instruments in *mestizo* culture is an idea drawn from occidental tradition. Of the indigenous wind instruments, the kena (end notched, 6 top, 1 back hole, approximately 13"-15"), often played in duos with parallel thirds, is the only one used frequently by mestizos. Interestingly, this small type of end-notched flute is used mainly in solo, informal contexts (e.g., while herding animals) by indigenous players, and is not considered particularly important.

Highland *mestizo* musical occasions range from stage and radio performance, to family and public Catholic fiestas. Mestizo musicians tend to be non- or part-time professional specialists. In *mestizo* Catholic fiestas, ensembles (mixed string and wind, or brass) are hired by rural town mestizos to supply the specific music for costumed dances often derived from Hispanic tradition. This music is known by the name of the dance accompanied: *Chuncho*s, *Qolla*s, etc. In addition, there are several major highland mestizo genres that are played generally. These include the *wayno* (moderate-fast duple meter, in two or three sections AA, BB, most often pentatonic), the *marinera* (moderate 6/8 meter, often diatonic, //:AA, BB, CC:// form), the *yaravi* (slow-lyrical, free or triple meter), *pas-odoble* and *muliza* (march-like). In contrast with the indigenous musical culture, these song or song-dance types, usually on light love themes, are free from specific contextual association.

In indigenous musical culture the value of repetition is linked to the idea that small or subtle changes (differentiating sections of a piece, songs, ensemble styles, etc.) are preferred over dramatic or large contrasts. In *mestizo* musical culture on the other hand, repetition is not favored to the same degree, and the principle of more obvious contrasts is taken from occidental culture. Hence, instead of performing a single piece for a long time, *mestizo* musicians often only perform three or four repetitions (music for costumed fiesta dancing is an exception). In addition, different genres are linked in medley for contrast. Thus, moderately paced marineras in 6/8 or slow lyrical yaravis are often followed with a *fuga* (a concluding song or section) of a faster *wayno* in duple meter. Another example of the use of obvious contrasts is in the mestizo charango tradition where strummed and plucked sections are alternated, whereas indigenous players only strum. So too, in mestizo ensembles, the mixing of various instrument types and the fact that different instruments take solo "breaks," provide contrasts of timbre. The very idea of using vocal and instrumental solos, stressing an individual's skill instead of the group "playing as one," is a mestizo-occidental feature.

Mestizo performance has been influenced in other major ways by occidental musical culture. A clearer, "purer" (less nasal, less airy, or with fewer overtones) vocal, wind, and string style is favored. A wide Western style vibrato distinguishes mestizo vocals, kena and string playing. Parallel thirds in melodic execution, and occidental triadic accompanying harmonies have replaced the unison, octaves or parallel 4ths/5ths characteristic of indigenous musical performance. More moderate pitch levels are also favored by mestizos who find the indigenous music too strident.

Urban-Andean Music

Beginning in the 1960s young people, largely from urban middle-class backgrounds in Andean cities, began to turn to features of rural highland music. In a sense this was part of the general trend of urban "folk music" revivals taking place in a number of western countries during this period. In contrast to the Chilean "nueva canción" movement with its more explicit political content, the urban-Andean style (see Wara 1984) diffused largely from La Paz, Bolivia, more directly involved musical/cultural/nationalistic identification with rural Andean society.

These ensembles combine a medium-sized *bombo* (double-headed drum) with guitars and nylon-stringed charangos. These instruments are used for rhythmic/harmonic accompaniment although the charango is usually allowed a melodic solo within a given performance. The lead melodic instrument of these urban "folk" groups is almost invariable the small kena, often alternated with solo zampoña (one player performs both panpipe rows). This kena style, beautiful in its own right, has more in common with European flute styles than with the Andean per se. It is characterized by a purer, less airy tone, wide vibrato, abundant trills and virtuostic playing. The panpipe, which exemplifies the Andean communal tradition par excellence, was turned into a solo instrument. A more staccato, less airy technique was developed (filling only the mouth of the tube instead of the traditional manner of filling the whole tube). On the charango, full triadic chords and tonal progressions are utilized when strummed, and single or double line solos are plucked replacing the indigenous style in which the melody is strummed on a single course with the rest of the open strings sounding. In addition, nylon strings are used instead of metal in order to achieve a "cleaner" sound preferred by urban-occidental aesthetics.

The urban Andean revivalist ensembles perform traditional pieces in *mestizo* genres such as the wayno, and the *cueca* (in 6/8, resembling the Peruvian *marinera*) as well as more indigenous forms. Original compositions based on *mestizo* genres are produced as well. The music is arranged for the stage in *peña*s ("folk" clubs) and for concerts in the larger cities such as La Paz, Cusco and Lima. These are the main performance contexts for this type of music whose audience in Peru is composed of the urban middle class and tourists. The arrangements feature smooth clear vocals, often with Western harmony, with solo instrumental "breaks," or an alternation of virtuostic solos on different instruments when vocals are absent.

In terms of musical form and values, this style is the most urban-occidental of the three types discussed here. European-based instrumental tone and performance techniques have replaced the Andean. Individual virtuosity and showmanship is stressed over "group blend." Contrast is stressed over repetition and more subtle changes. Urban professional-stage performance has replaced community ceremonies and fiestas in the indigenous context, as well as Catholic town and family fiestas among mestizos (although mestizos also perform on stage). The urban-Andean style, however, is the most immediately appealing to urban and non-Andean audiences, and serves as a good entrance into the world of more traditional styles. Just as the Kingston Trio and Peter, Paul and Mary led interested North Americans back to the roots of Appalachian and southern black traditional music, urban-Andean performers such as Savia Andina and Uña Ramos may well lead to a discovery of the incredible wealth and beauty of music still performed throughout the rural Andean highlands.

Tom Turino is presently on the faculty of the Music Department at the University of Illinois Champagne-Urbana. He has done extensive field work in the Andean region of Peru, supported in part by a Fulbright Research Fellowship.

Further Readings:

Garcilaso de la Vega. *Comentarios Reales de los Incas.* (Cusco: Universidad del Cusco, 1960).

Guaman Poma de Ayala, Felipe. *Nueva Cronica y Buen Gobierno.* (Lima: IEP, 1980).

Haeberli, Joerg. "Twelve Nasca Panpipes: A Study," *Ethnomusicology* 23(1):57-73, 1979.

Rossell Castro, P. *Arqueologia Sur del Peru.* (Lima: Editores Universo S.A., 1977).

Stevenson, Robert. *Music in Aztec and Inca Territory.* (Berkeley: University of California Press, 1968).

Turino, Thomas. "The Urban Mestizo Charango Tradition in Southern Peru: A Statement of Shifting Identity," *Ethnomusicology* 28(2):253-270, 1984.

"The Charango and the Sirena: Music, Magic and the Power of Love," *Latin American Music Review* 4(1):81-119, 1983.

Wara Cespedes, Gilka. "New Currents in Musica Folklorica in La Paz, Bolivia," *Latin American Music Review* 5(2):217-242, 1984.

VOICES OF THE AMERICAS 1986 CONCERT SERIES
Washington Square Church, N.Y.C.

Picking the Piedmont Blues
January 24 and 25
John Cephas and Phil Wiggins
John Jackson
John Dee Holeman

The Black Gospel Tradition
February 1
The Fairfield Four
The Faithful Harmonizers
Mt. Zion Pentecostal Young People's Choir

Music of Argentina and Colombia
February 8
Los Troveros Cuyanos
Aires Colombianos

Music and Dance of Haiti and Cuba
February 14
La Troupe Makandal
Orlando "Puntilla" Rios and Nueva Generacion

A cappella—Sacred and Secular
March 1
The Badgett Sisters
New Emage

Music and Dance of Puerto Rico
March 8
Los Pleneros de la 21
Israel Berrios y El Quinteto Criollo

Cajun Music and the Roots of Zydeco
March 14 and 15
Alphonse "Boisec" Ardoin and Canray Fontenot
Beausoleil

Music of Peru and the High Andes
March 22
Tahuantinsuyo
Fabian Mozaurieta

Blues from the Delta to Chicago
April 11 and 12
James 'Son' Thomas
Cedell Davis
Carey Bell Blues Band

Mexican Vocal Traditions
April 19
Lydia Mendoza
Los Pregoneros Del Puerto

Cowboy Songs and Western Swing
April 26
Glenn Ohrlin
Junior Daugherty

Music and Dance of Honduras and Belize
May 3
Garifuna Folk Dance Ensemble

Music of the Bolivian Andes
May 9
Sukay

The Roots of Country Music
May 10
Ola Belle and Bud Reed
Bessie Eldreth
The Whitstein Brothers

Music of the Iroquois and Pan Indian Dance
May 31
The Standing Arrow Singers

*also included on the Voices of the Americas cassette series are Dennis McGee and Sady Courville who performed with Beausoleil on November 7, 1986

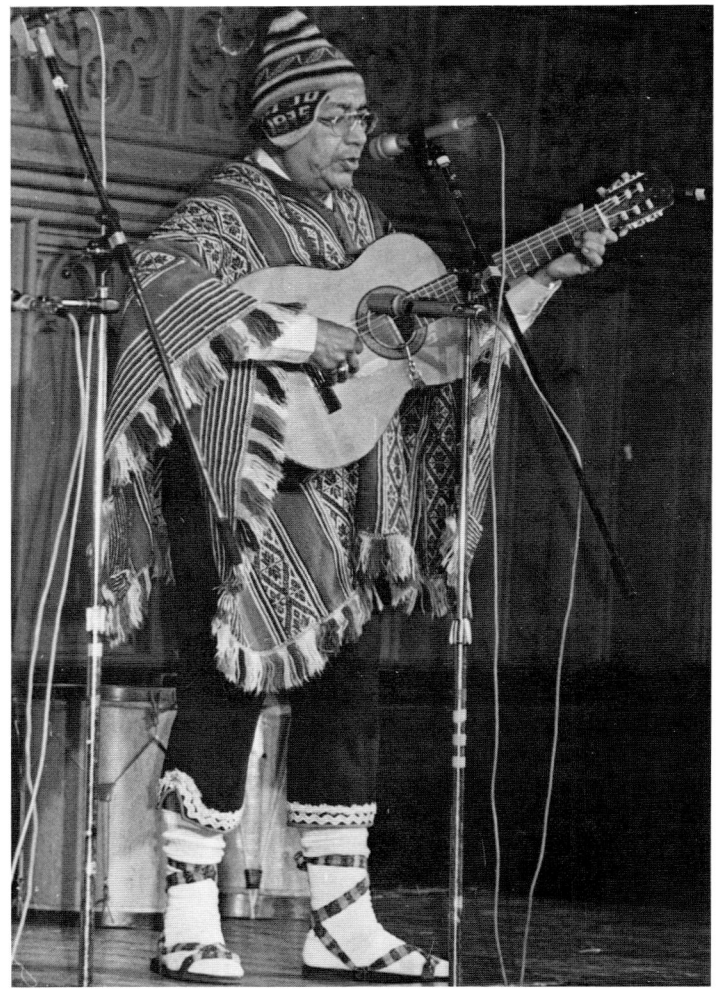

Fabian Mozaurieta singing a Peruvian *Huayno*.

Voices of the Americas Biographies

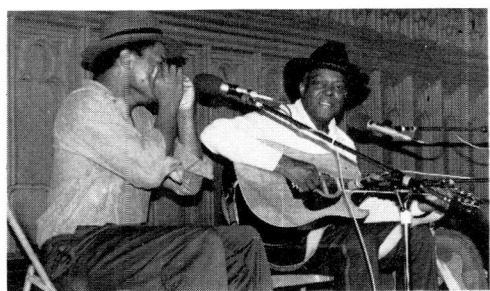

"Bowling Green" John Cephas and Phil Wiggins, veterans of Big Chief Ellis' Barrelhouse Rockers, have been playing together since 1977. Cephas was born and reared in the small Virginia town of Bowling Green. At the age of ten he began playing guitar under the tutelage of his aunt and several local blues musicians. His intricate finger picking style and smooth vocals reflect the influence of recordings by Piedmont masters such as Gary Davis and Blind Boy Fuller. Phil Wiggins, born in Washington, DC, in 1954, learned his innovative harmonica styles from recordings of Hammie Nixon, Big Walter Horton, Sonny Boy Williamson, and other blues harp virtuosos. The duo's lively performances are squarely in the tradition of blues masters Sonny Terry and Brownie McGee.

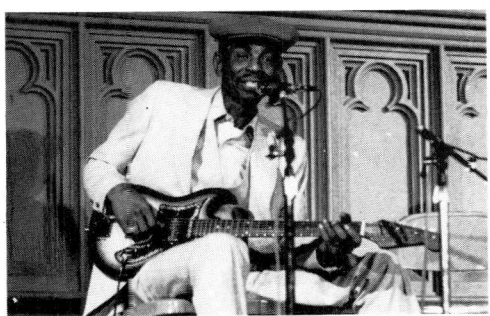

Born in Orange County, North Carolina, **John Dee Holeman** began picking the guitar at the age of 14, learning Piedmont standards from his uncle and cousin, as well as other regional and national styles that were readily available on record. At the age of 25 he moved to Durham and began playing electric guitar. His smooth vocal style combined with his ability to play traditional pieces as well as more recent popular boogies made him a favorite at house parties and clubs.

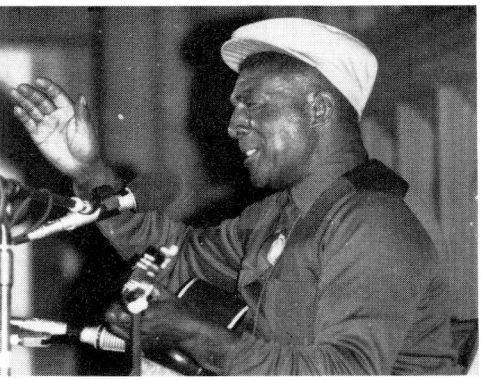

John Jackson, born in Rappahannock County, Virginia in 1924, epitomizes the smooth swing of the Piedmont blues with his lilting, ragtime-influenced picking style. While growing up on a plantation he absorbed musical elements from his father, who played guitar and banjo and sang for house parties, and his mother, who played accordion and sang church songs and spirituals. His smooth vocal style also reflects the influence of white country singers like Jimmie Rodgers, the Carter Family, and the Delmore Brothers, whom he heard on radio and early hillbilly recordings. An extremely versatile musician, Jackson is one of the few remaining bluesmen who doubles on guitar and banjo.

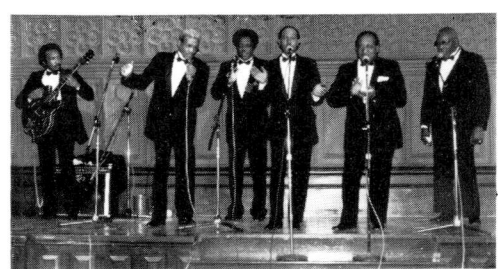

The **Fairfield Four** is one of the oldest and most respected gospel quartets in the country today. Formed in 1921 by a group of youngsters from Nashville's Fairfield Baptist Church, the Fairfield Four broadcast regularly on Nashville's prestigious WLAC during the 1930s, and enjoyed a lucrative recording and touring career during the 1940s and early 1950s. After a twenty year hiatus, the group was reorganized in 1980, and today includes singers James Hill (baritone and bass) and Isaac "Dickie" Freeman (bass), who were with the group in the 1940s. They are joined by lead singer Lawrence Richardson, tenor singer Wilson Waters, and guitarist Lewis McBride. The Fairfield's tight, four-part harmony singing and syncopated rhythmic pulse are suggestive of the older jubilee style quartets, while Richardson's improvised, preaching style lead vocals reflect a more recent, post-War approach to gospel quartet singing.

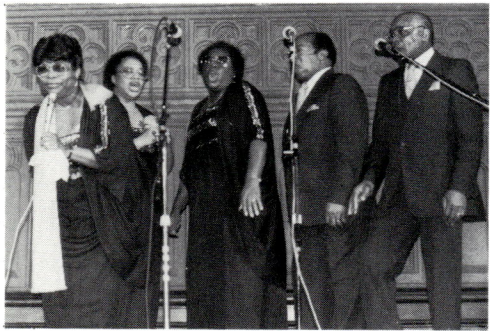

Led by Reverend Vernella Kelly, the **Faithful Harmonizers** have been serving churches throughout the New York metropolitan area for nearly forty years. The group, which today includes William Ray, Geneva Ray, Wilburt Huntly, and Clara Makey, features traditional a cappella arrangements of many old church songs and gospel standards. Their unique blend of male and female voices along with a moving bass vocal produces a richly textured sound that is reminiscent of the older jubilee choirs and quartets. Reverend Kelly's fiery lead vocals and spirit-induced testimonies suggest the influence of more modern gospel singing.

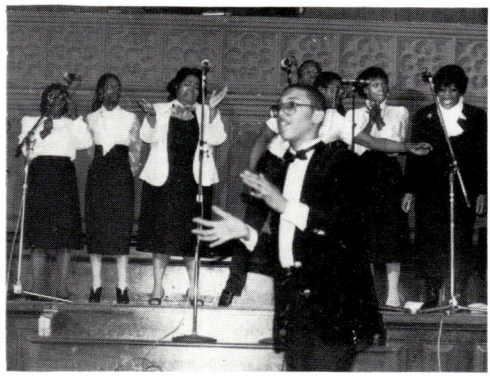

Based at Brooklyn's Mt. Zion Pentecostal Church, **The Mt. Zion Penetecostal Young**

People's Choir includes some of New York's most exciting young gospel performers. The group sings regularly at their home church's Sunday morning services, and is often invited to perform at neighboring churches on Sunday afternoon and evening programs. Led by arranger/writer Paul Evans, the 14-voice ensemble with drum and keyboard accompaniment renders modern gospel arrangements of older hymns and church songs as well as contemporary gospel and original compositions. Their captivating sound reflects the diverse influences of European choral music, African-American jazz, and the rhythmic music of the black Pentecostal church.

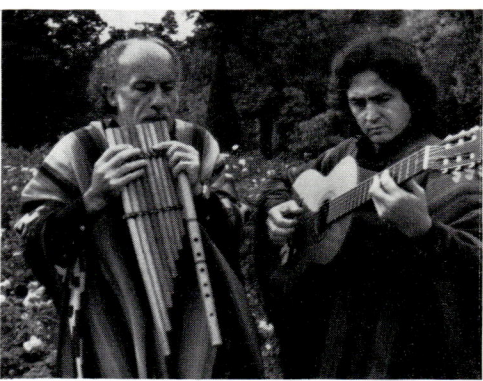

Los Troveros Cuyanos is an Inca word meaning "the messengers of peace, news, and harmony." Composed of Rodolfo Dalera and Francisco Navarro, the group has gained an international reputation for their sensitive renditions of the music of their native Argentina. They interpret a number of Spanish-derived song forms from the lowland regions of Argentina including *chacarera*, *tonada*, and *zamba*. In keeping with tradition, these songs are arranged for dual vocals with guitar accompaniment. They also incorporate flutes, panpipes, and *charango* from the southern Andes region of Argentina into their performances.

Aires Colombianos is dedicated to performing traditional Colombian Music, a mestizo style that combines aspects of Spanish heritage with indigenous Native American rhythms and melodies. The group, composed of Maria Olga Pineros, Jose E. Hernandez, Guillermo Gaviria, features both the music of the Andes with the *Bambuco* as its most representative expression and that of the plains with the *Jorop* as its most characteristic song style. Besides its fine harmony singing, the group plays an assortment of flutes, percussion, and string instruments.

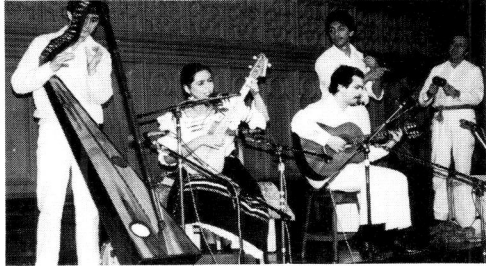

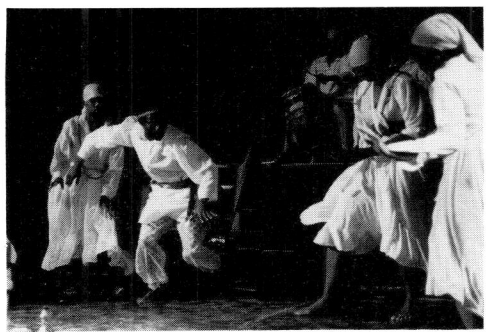

La Troupe Makandal was organized in 1973 in Belair, a small community in Port-au-Prince, Haiti. In 1981 they re-formed in New York City, under the leadership of master drummer Frisner Augustin. They specialize in the sacred music and dance traditions of Haiti, including the ceremonial Vodoun music and the *rara* processionals associated with Holy Week celebrations. Their performances at schools, museums, and other cultural organizations throughout the New York City metropolitan area have done much to preserve and perpetuate these traditions.

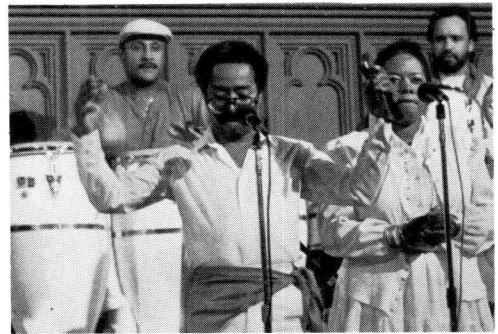

Acknowledged in his native Cuba as a master *bata* drummer, **Orlando "Puntilla" Rios** emigrated to the United States in 1981.

After settling in New York City he organized **Nueva Generacion,** a group of Cuban-Americans dedicated to the preservation and presentation of the sacred music and dance of *Santeria*, as well as the various secular forms of *rumba*. The group consists of Orlando Rios (lead vocals), Oscar Gonzales (vocals, shekere), Olufemi Mitchell (vocals, shekere), Anthony Carrillo (bata drum), Felix Sanbria (bata drum), Daniel Ponce (conga drum), Carlos Cordova (trap drums), Xiomara Rodriguez (dance and vocals), Rita Masoa (dance and vocals), and Freddy Alvares (dance and vocals).

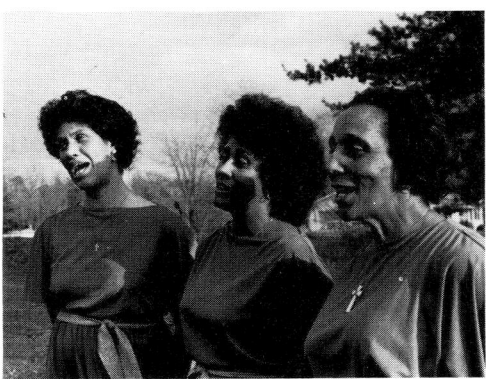

The **Badgett Sisters** are among the last of the close-harmony, a cappella sacred groups that still sing in the jubilee and harmonizing styles commonly associated with the pre-War quartet tradition. Cleonia Badgett Graves (lead and tenor), Celestar Badgett Sellars (tenor and lead), and Connie Badgett Steadman (alto) are three sisters from the heart of North Carolina tobacco country who have performed together since 1945 when their father first taught them the basics of part singing. They are members of the Graves Chapel Baptist Church in Yanceyville and sing primarily for local church and school.

New Emage welds together one of the best urban folk traditions—street corner harmonizing. Hailing from Philadelphia, which during the 1950s hosted one of the nation's most influential communities of doo-wop singers, New Emage's members all began singing on street corners where they gathered informally to harmonize R&B standards. Since organizing as a group in the late 1970s, they have appeared at many festivals, including the Festival of American Folklife at the Smithsonian Institution, and toured the Caribbean. New Emage is comprised of Ricardo Rose, Andrew Rose, Darrall Campbell, Anthony Williams and Al Williams.

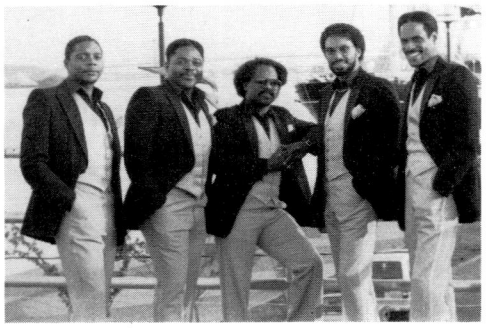

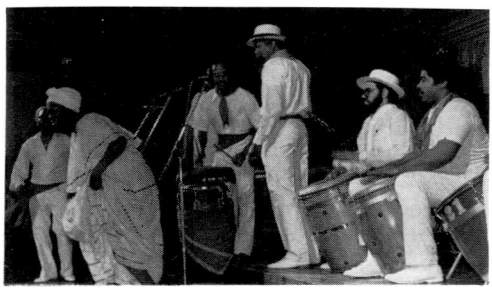

Los Pleneros de la 21 takes its name from *Parada 21* (Bus Stop #21), a gathering place in the predominantly black neighborhood in the Santurce sector of San Juan. Formed in 1983 by Juan Gutierrez, this New York based group of singers, dancers, and drummers includes many of the older masters of *bamba* and *plena* who grew up performing within their communities in Puerto Rico. The group's frequent festival and concert appearances have led to an increased awareness of traditional Puerto Rican music and dance forms within New York City's Latin Community. Los Pleneros consists of Juan Gutierrez (percussion), Paco Rivera (dance and lead vocal), Sammy Tanco (lead vocal), Pable Ortiz (lead vocal), Eugenia Ramos (dance and percussion), Tito Cepeda (percussion), Michael Carrillo (percussion), Benjamin Flores (percussion), Edgardo Miranda (cuatro), and Donald Nicks (bass).

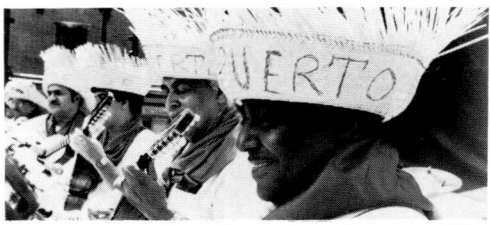

Panos Papanicolaon—Courtesy of EFAC

El Quinteto Criollo was formed in 1952 by the well known Puerto Rican guitarist **Israel Berrios,** in order to perpetuate Puerto Rico's various Spanish derived vocal and instrumental traditions known as *jibaro* music. The group consist of Israel Berrios (guitar and vocals), Tobeta Modina (vocals), Mario Hernandez (guitar), Pepe Roman (percussion), and Miguel Carrillo (trumpet).

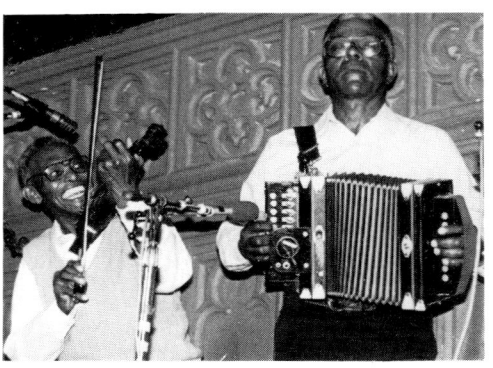

Reared in an environment rich in traditional Louisiana blues and dance music, **Alphonse 'Boisec' Ardoin** and **Canray Fontenot** are the finest living exponents of early black Creole music. Born in l'Anse de 'Prien Noir in 1916, Ardoin learned to play accordion from his older cousin, the legendary Amede Ardoin, the first Creole performer to make commercial recordings. Fontenot, a native of l'Anse des Rougeaux, was born into a musical family in 1918. His father, Adam Fontenot, and older cousin, Freeman Fontenot, were renowed accordionists, but young Canray chose to take up the fiddle at the age of eleven, learning from his cousin, Douglas Belair, and other community musicians. Ardoin and Fontenot have been playing together in house parties and dance halls across rural Louisiana since the late 1930s, and in the past twenty years have performed at festivals throughout the United States, Canada, and Europe.

Beausoleil, named after the Acadian rebel leader Beausoleil Broussard, is one of today's most influential forces in the revival of French Louisiana music. Based in Lafayette, Louisiana, the group was formed in 1975 by Michael Doucet, an active promoter of Cajun music and culture. In researching the roots of his music, Doucet studied with the most esteemed practitioners of the older Cajun and black Creole styles including Dennis McGee, the Balfa Brothers, Canray

Fontenot, and Hector Duhan. Beausoleil is composed of Michael Doucet (fiddle and vocals), Errol Verret (accordion), David Doucet (guitar and vocals), Billy Ware (*frottoir*—washboard and *petit fer*—triangle), Tommy Comeaux (mandolin), and Tommy Alessi (drums).

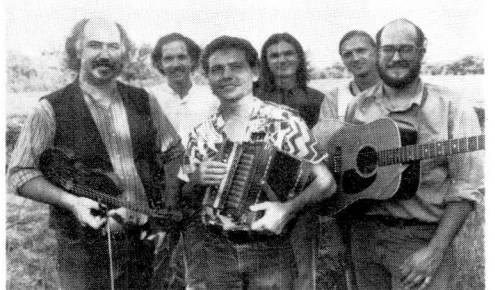

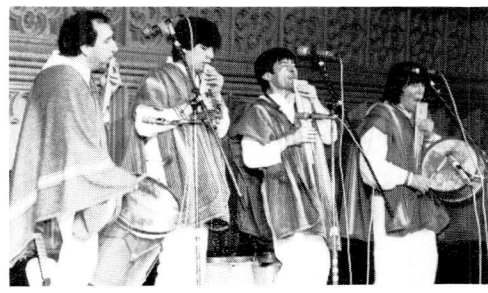

Tahuantinsuyo takes its name from the Quechua word that the Incas used to describe their empire, literally "the four corners of the world." Dedicated to the preservation and presentation of the traditional music of the high Andes, group members have spent years researching the culture and recreating the authentic vocal and instrumental styles of the region. Currently based in Queens, New York City, the group has toured extensively throughout North and South America. Organized in 1974, Tahuantinsuyo presently consists of founding members Pepe Santana and Guillermo Guerrero, natives of Ecuador and Peru respectively, and Peruvian born emigrants Alcides Loza and Isaac Lopez.

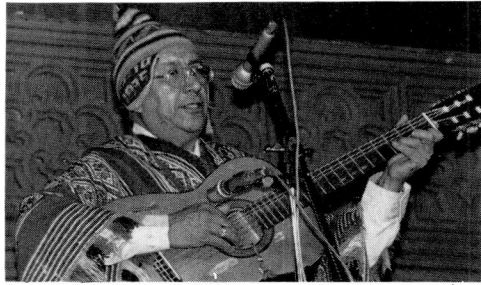

Fabian Mozaurita, a native of Cotahuasi, Peru, immigrated to the United States in 1974. Acknowledged as an authentic interpreter of the traditional Peruvian Mestizo song form known as *huayno*, he sings in Quechua and Spanish, accompanying himself on guitar and *charango*. Since settling in New York City he has performed at numerous folk festivals and concerts throughout the metropolitan area.

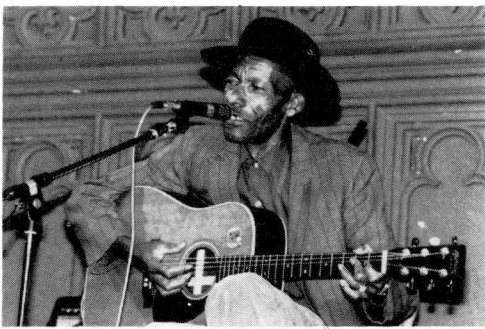

Born and reared on a farm near Eden in the Mississippi Delta county of Yazoo, **James "Son" Thomas** learned the rudiments of Delta blues guitar from his Uncle, Joe Cooper. Recordings of early Delta blues artists including Sonny Boy Williams, Arthur "Big Boy" Crudup, and Elmore James also exerted strong influences on his style. For years he played in small cafes and juke joints throughout the Leland/Greenville region of Mississippi, and more recently has found an appreciative audience on folk festival circuits throughout the United States and Europe. His hard-edged guitar and swooping vocals harken back to the earlier Delta styles.

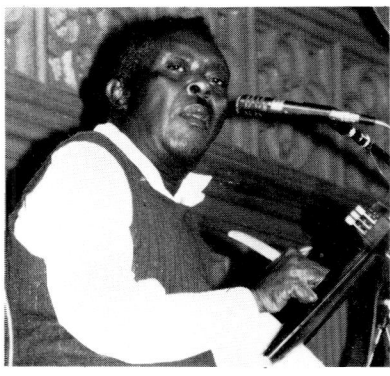

Cedell Davis was born in Helena, an important blues center in the northern Delta region of Arkansas. Stricken by polio as a child, he developed an innovative guitar style by sliding a knife across the upper strings with his right hand. The use of glass and metal slides is one of the hallmarks of the Delta style, as is Davis' raspy, moaning vocal delivery. Davis played with the legendary Robert Nighthawk during the 1940s, and eventually moved to Pine Bluff, Arkansas, where he continues to perform and tour.

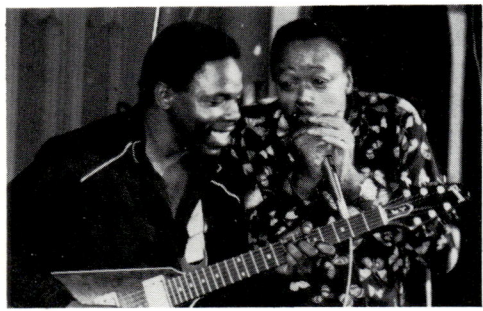

The Carey Bell Blues Band, formed in 1979 by blues harpist Carey Bell Harrington, is currently one of Chicago's leading blues acts. Born in 1936 in Macon, Mississippi, Bell began playing harmonica with his step father, piano player and bluesman Lovey Lee. At the age of nineteen, Bell came north to Chicago to play with the Lovey Lee Blues Band, and later went on to perform and record with such legendary figures as Muddy Waters, Howlin' Wolf, Willie Dixon, Sonny Boy Williams, and Honey Boy Edwards. The senior Bell is currently joined by his son, Lurrie Bell, who has been acclaimed as one of the finest guitarists in the new generation of Chicago bluesmen. Drummer Dino Davies and bassist Michael Morrison fill out the ensemble. Bell's distinctive harp style propels the band forward with a sound personifying the contemporary Chicago blues scene.

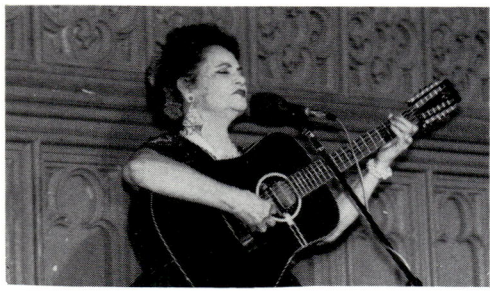

The legendary **Lydia Mendoza**, known as "La Alondra de la Frontera" (Songbird of the Border), has been one of the leading exponents of Mexican-American Norteno music since the 1920s. She was born in Houston in 1916 to a family boasting several generations of singers and musicians. By the age of nine she was proficient on the guitar, violin and mandolin and began travelling with her father, mother and sister as an integral part of the Carta Blance Quartet. She made her first recordings with her family in 1928 and made her first solo records on Bluebird in 1934, accompanying herself on 12-string guitar. She had an active and successful recording and concert career in the 1930s, becoming immensely popular in southern Texas and northern Mexico. She continued to record following World War II, and during the past decade reestablished her touring career through numerous appearances at folk festivals across the United States.

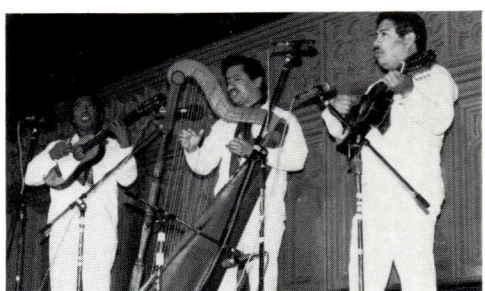

Los Pregoneros del Puerto is led by Jose Gutierrez, a native of La Costa De La Palma, in the heart of Mexico's jarocho country near the port of Veracruz. He performs all the standard jarocho instruments —the *arpa*, the 36-string Mexican harp; the *requinto*, a 4-string guitar; and the *jarana*, an 8-string guitar—and is a superb vocal and instrumental improvisor. Gutierrez is joined by Manuel Vasquez and Gonzalo Mata. Together the trio has been performing at folk festivals and universities throughout the United States for the past six years.

Born in Minneapolis in 1925, **Glenn Ohrlin** has been a cowboy virtually all his life. At the age of 16, two years after his family had moved to California, he ran off to Nevada to work as a ranch hand and ride in the rodeo circuit. For the past twenty years he has lived on his own ranch in Stone County, Arkansas. Ohrlin has spent his entire life absorbing cowboy folklore, and today is a wellspring of traditional cowboy songs, poetry, and stories. His diverse repertoire also includes older ballads, sentimental songs, bawdy ditties, and country western favorites. Aside from his superb talents as a singer and story teller, Ohrlin has published an important collection of cowboy songs entitled *Hell-Bound Train* (University of Illinois Press).

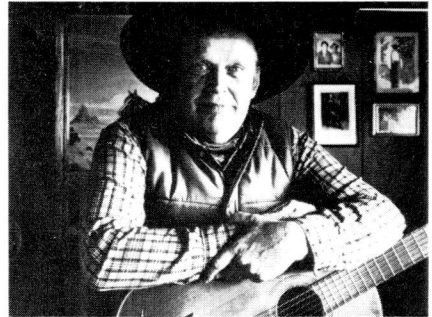

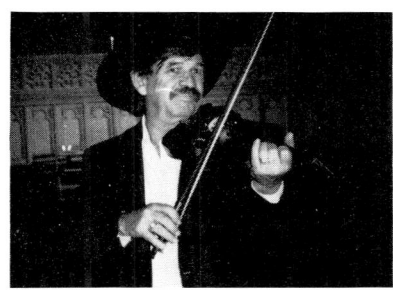

Junior Daugherty was brought up in a ranching and blacksmithing family in southern New Mexico. At the age of eight he was singing and playing backup guitar for his grandfather, a blacksmith and well respected local fiddler. Young Junior eventually took up the fiddle, going on to win numerous fiddle championships and earning himself the reputation of one of America's top country fiddlers. His playing reflects the influence of the western swing music popularized by artists such as Bob Wills in the 1930s, as well as traditional bluegrass and more contemporary country styles. He croons cowboy and country songs in a rich baritone voice that never fails to stir the listener's sentiments. Daugherty is joined by fiddler Julie Kitzenberger.

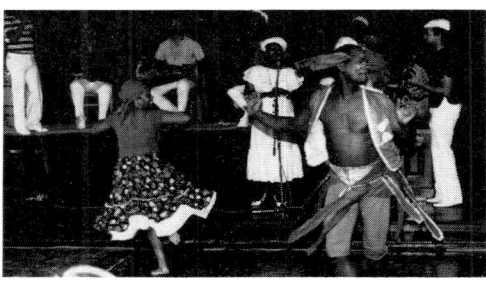

The Garifuna Folk Dance Ensemble, led by John Mariano, consists of singers, dancers, and percussionists who have migrated to New York city from Belize, Honduras, and Guatemala. They perform the traditional songs and dances of the Garifuna, a group of Afro-Caribbean people descended from shipwrecked and runaway slaves and Carib Indians who settled in the coastal regions of Central America during the eighteenth century. Their music is a rich and creative amalgam of West African, Carib Indian, and European cultural traditions.

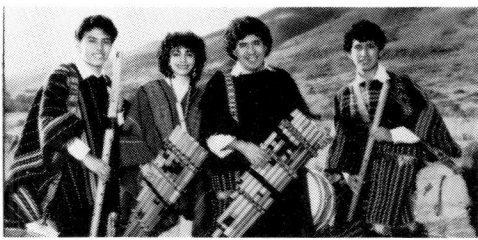

Sukay, which in Quechua means "to open up the earth and prepare it for planting," is a San Franciso based quartet that performs traditional and contemporary vocal and instrumental music of the Andes. Founded in 1978 by Quentin Howard, a native of Brooklyn, New York, other members of the group include Carlos Crespo and Mario Lino of Bolivia, and Omar Sepulveda from Chile. This recording features their interpretation of traditional Bolivian songs as well as contemporary songs in the traditional style written by Carlos Crespo.

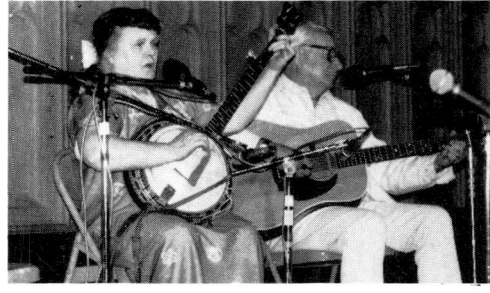

Performances by **Ola Belle** and **Bud Reed** are reminiscent of the early hillbilly sounds of the 1920s and 1930s. Ola Belle Reed was born in Ashe County, North Carolina, where she learned to play the traditional Appalachian down picking/strumming banjo style known as "clawhammer." There she also developed a broad repertoire of traditional songs learned primarily from her grandmother and her mother, Ella Mae Osborne Campbell. During the Depression her family left North Carolina and eventually settled in Maryland, where Ola Belle joined the North Carolina Ridge Runners of York Lynn, Delaware, one of the area's earliest hillbilly bands. In 1949 she married Bud Reed, a native of Maryland who had been playing and singing at community dances for many years. During the 1950s the Reeds operated the New River Ranch, near Rising Sun, Maryland, and introduced many leading country artists to northern audiences. Ola Belle and her brother, Alex, hosted a popular radio program during the 1950s and early 1960s that was influential in the ensuing folk music revival. Since the mid-1960s Ola Belle and Bud Reed have appeared at folk festivals throughout the United States and Canada.

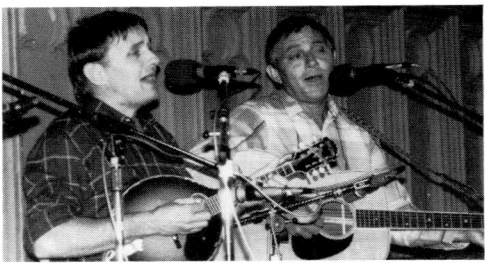

The **Whitstein Brothers,** of Pineville, Louisiana, are carrying on the venerable tradition of brother duos that reached its height of popularity in country music during the 1930s and 1940s. Their tight harmony renditions of love songs, country classics, and gospel numbers are reminiscent of the sounds of such influential groups as the Blue Sky Boys and the Delmore Brothers. Bob (mandolin) and Charles (guitar) Whitstein were strongly influenced by their father, R.G. Whitstein, who was an accomplished guitarist, fiddler, and singer, and who hosted a weekly country radio show in Pineville. The young Whitsteins performed primarily in dances, schools, and churches in central Louisiana, and in 1964 appeared on Nashville's Grand Old Opry. In recent years they have found a new and appreciative audience on the folk festival circuit.

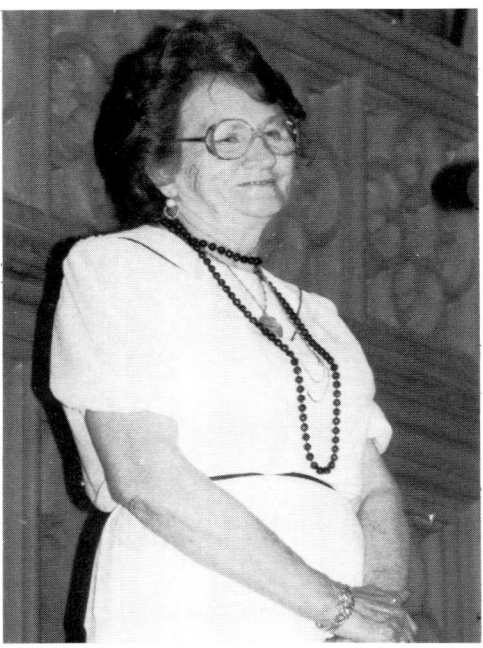

Singer **Bessie Eldreth** was born in Ashe County, North Carolina, in 1913. Reared in a musical family, her mother and grandmother were outstanding ballad singers and her father was an accomplished fiddler and banjo player. She learned her diverse repertoire of sacred and secular songs from family, friends, and fellow church-goers. Until recently her singing was limited to home and church settings within her community, but in the past few years she has brought her traditional mountain style balladry to appreciative audiences at larger folk festivals.

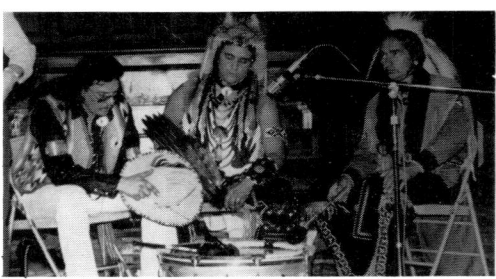

The Standing Arrow Singers and Dancers hail from Akwesasne, the Mohawk reservation on the New York/Canadian border. Their broad repertoire consists of the social dance music of the Iroquois (Mohawk, Seneca, Cayuga, Onondaga, Onedia and Tuscarora) as well as other Native American nations. The Standing Arrow Singers and Dancers are named after the late Mohawk elder, Frank "Standing Arrow" Thomas, who instilled in his family a great knowledge and pride in their own and other Native American cultures. They have performed at inter-tribal Pow-Wows and other cultural events throughout the United States and Canada.

Born in 1893, **Dennis McGee** learned to play fiddle from his father, grandfather, uncles, and other community members in l'Anse des Rougeaux, near Eunice, Louisiana. He has been playing for more than seventy-five years, mostly with brother-in-law **Sady Courville.** Their twin-fiddling provides a direct link to nineteenth century styles that pre-date the advent of the accordion in Cajun music. McGee and Courville were among the first South Louisiana musicians to make commercial records in the late 1920s, and their initial recordings—such as "Ma Chere Bebe Creole"—provide a vital documentation of early Cajun fiddling. Among the last bearers of their venerable tradition, McGee and Courville have been at the forefront of the Cajun music revival through their numerous festival and concert performances during the past twenty-five years.

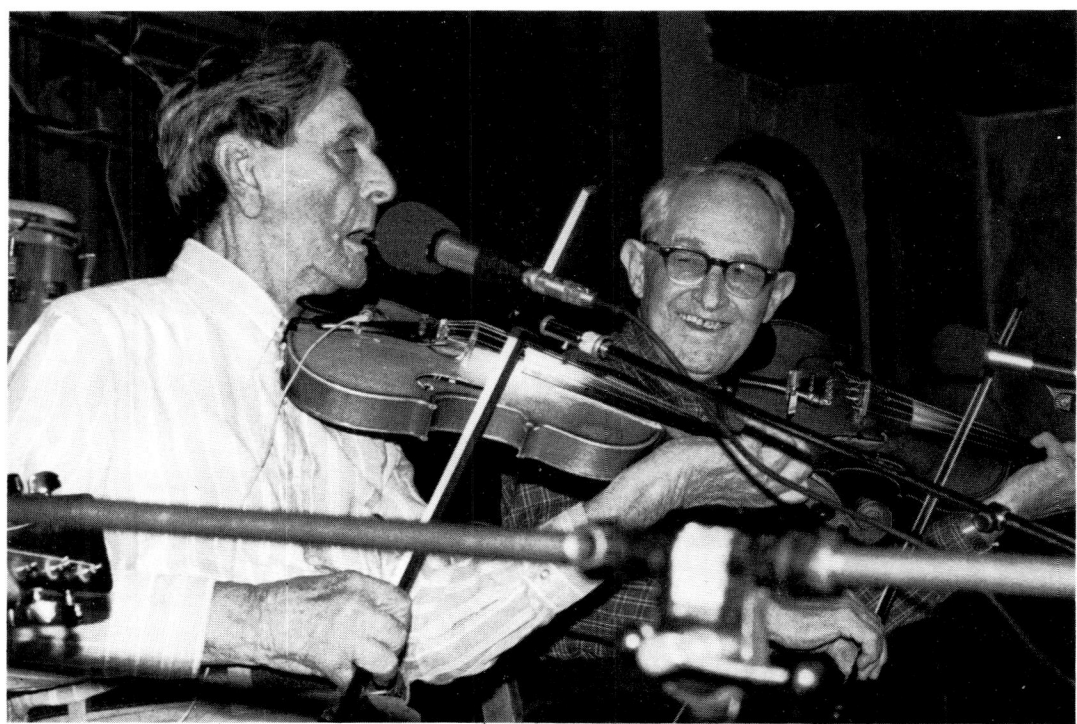

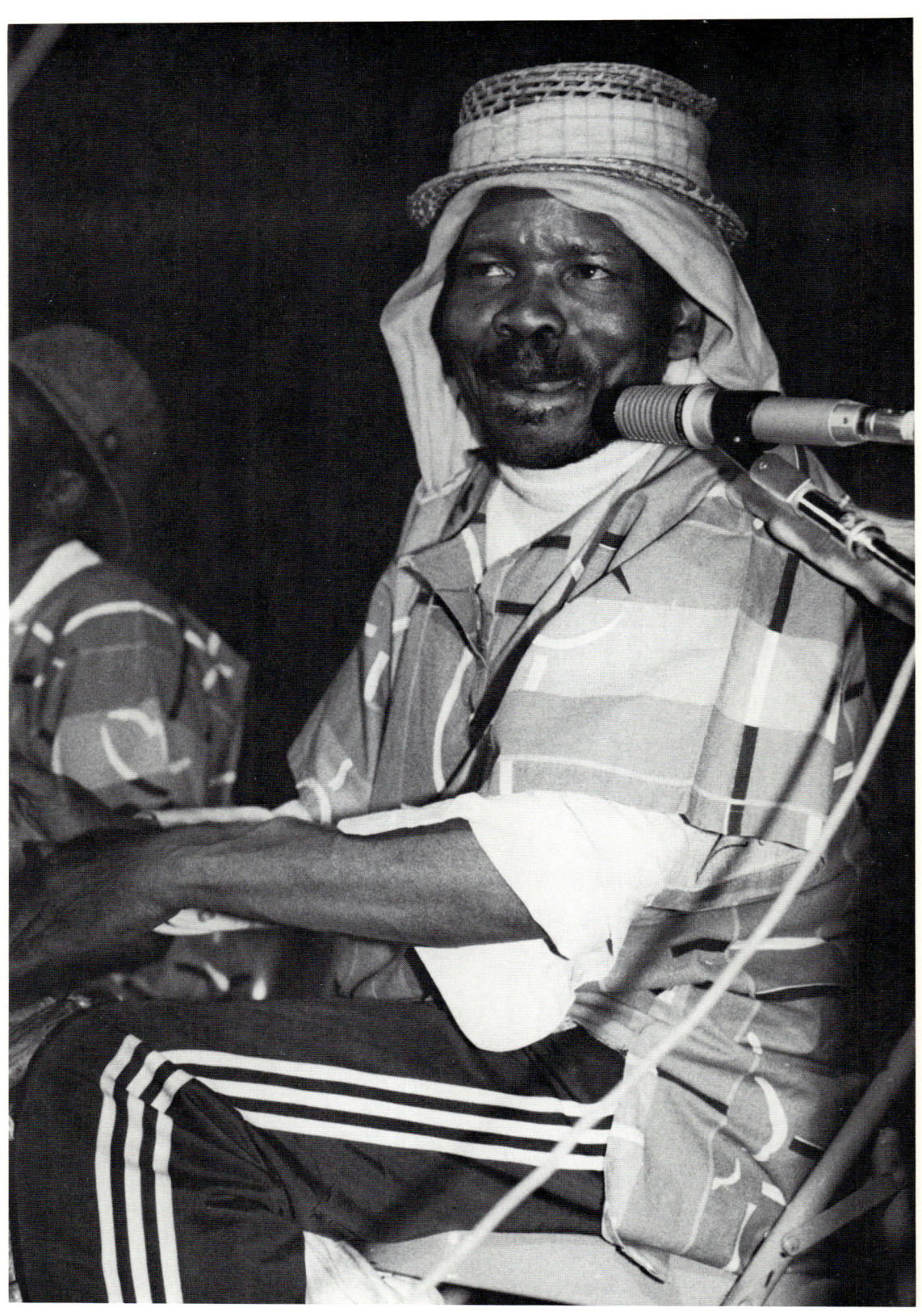
John Mariano leader of the Garifuna Folk Dance Ensemble.

Discography by Ray Allen

Native American

"Indian Music of the Southwest." Recording and booklet compiled by Laura Boulton, Folkways Records FW-8850, 1957.

"Iroquois Social Dance Songs." Iroqrafts QC-727, 1969.

"Night and Daylight Yeibichai." Compiled by Tony Isaacs, Indian House IH-1502, 1968.

"Music of the Sioux and the Navajo." Recordings and booklet compiled by Williard Rhodes, Folkways Records FE-4401, 1949.

Blues

"Blues Roots/Mississippi." Folkways RBF-14. (Includes selections of early Mississippi blues by Tommy Johnson, Robert Johnson, Joe Williams, others.)

"Ain't Gonna Rain No More." Recordings and annotated notes compiled by Christopher Lornell, Rounder Records RR-2016. (Includes field recordings of Piedmont, North Carolina pre-blues string band and ragtime music.)

"Roots of the Blues." Recordings and annotated notes by Alan Lomax, New World Records NW-252. (Field recordings from northern Mississippi.)

"Blind Blake Volume II: Search Warrant Blues." Biograph BLP-12023. (Essential early Piedmont country blues.)

"Muddy Waters: Sail On." Chess-1539. (Classic early Chicago urban blues.)

"B.B. King: Live at the Regal." ABCS-724. (Outstanding live urban blues.)

Country

"Smithsonian Collection of Classic Country Music." Recordings and booklet compiled by Bill Malone, Smithsonian Institution, 1981. (eight lp set includes outstanding country recordings from 1921 through the early 1970s.)

"Anthology of American Folk Music." Recording and booklet compiled by Harry Smith, Folkways Records, FA-2951-53. (Includes early recordings of country ballads and hillbilly music, as well as a smattering of blues, gospel, and cajun material).

"Old-Time Southern Dance Music—Volumes I and II." Old-Timey Records, OT-100 and 101. (Early fiddle/banjo/guitar recordings including selections by Eck Robertson, Gid Tanner and the Skillet Lickers, Riley Pucket, Arthur Smith, others.)

"Western Swing." Old-Timey Records, OT-105. (Includes classic recordings by Bob Wills, Milton Brown, the Light Crust Dough Boys, others.)

"The Carter Family on Border Radio." John Edwards Memorial Foundation, JEMF-101. (Early recordings of classic mountain ballads and lyrical songs by the best known of the early hillbilly artists.)

African-American Gospel

"An Introduction to Gospel Song." Recordings and annotated notes compiled by Samuel Charters, Folkways Records, RBF-5, 1962. (Includes selections by the Fisk University Jubilee Quartet, Reverend J.M. Gates and Congregation, Ernistine Washington, the Spirit of Memphis, others.)

"Father and Sons." Recordings and annotated notes compiled by Tony Heilbut, SpiritFeel Records (Shanachie), SF1001, 1986. (Includes selections by the Soul Stirrers, the 5 Blind Boys of Mississippi, and the Nightingales.)

"Birmingham Quartet Anthology, 1926-1953." Recordings and booklet compiled by Doug Seroff, Chanka Lanka Records, CL-144,001/002, 1980. (Includes selections by the Birmingham Jubilee Singers, the Famous Blue Jay Singers, The Heavenly Gospel Singers, others.)

"Jubilee To Gospel: A Selection of Commercially Recorded Black Religious Music, 1921-1953." Recordings and booklet compiled by William Tallmadge, John Edwards Memorial Foundaiton, JEMF-108, 1980. (Includes selections by the Fisk Jubilee Singers, Wings Over Jordan Choir, the Fairfield Four, the Golden Gate Quartet, others.)

"The Gospel Sound, Volumes I and II." Compiled by Tony Heilbut, Columbia G-31595. (Includes selections by Mahalia Jackson, Dorothy Love Coats, the Golden Gate Quartet, the Dixie Hummingbirds, others.)

"James Cleveland Sings with the World's Greatest Gospel Choirs." Savoy Records, SGL-7059.

Cuban/Puerto Rican

"*Caliente* = Hot, Puerto Rican and Cuban Musical Expression in New York City." Recordings and booklet compiled by Roberta Singer and Robert Friedman, New World Records-NW 224, 1977. (Outstanding field recordings of traditional *bomba, plena, son, Santeria, rumba,* and *jibaro* music.)

"Concepts on Unity—*Grupo Folklorico y Experimental Nueva Yorgyino.*" Salsoul 2-400. (More exemplary recordings of traditional Cuban and Puerto Rican music performed by New York City's leading Latin musicians.)

"Milton Cardonia—*Bembe.*" American Clave 10014, 1986. (Traditional Afro-Cuban chanting and drumming from *Santeria* ceremonies).

"Folksongs of Puerto Rico." Recordings and booklet compiled by Henrietta Yurchenco, Folkways Records, Asch Mankind Series, 1971.

"*Exitos De Arsenio Rodriguez and Su Conjunto.*" Tropical Records TRLP-5005. (Afro-Cuban *mambo* and other dance rhythms performed by master percussionist and *tres* player Arsenio Rodriguez and his band.)

"Mucho Macho Machito and his Afro-Cuban Salseros." Pablo Records 2625 712, 1978. (Vintage late 1940s' recordings of pre-salsa, Afro-Cuban jazz by Machito, the master of the idiom.)

Cajun/Creole

"Louisiana French Cajun Music From the South West Prairies, Volumes 1 and 2." Rounder Records RR-6001&2. (Includes selections by Balfa Brothers, Canray Fontenot, Alphonse Ardoin, others.)

"Louisiana Cajun Music, Volumes 1-5." Old Timey Records, OT-108-111, 114. (Includes re-issues of definitive Cajun recordings from the 1920s through the 1950s.)

"The Early Recordings of Dennis McGee: Morning Star 45002. (Includes re-issues of McGee's seminal late 1920s and 1930s recordings with Sady Courville and Ernest Fruge.)

"*Zodico:* Louisiana Creole Music." Recordings and booklet compiled by Nick Spitzer, Rounder Records, RR-6009, 1977. (Field recordings of outstanding black Creole music including selections by Bebe and Eraste Carriere, the Lawtell Playboys, others.)

"*Boisec—La Musique Creole.*" Arhoolie 1070. (Accordion/fiddle Creole music by Alphonse Ardoin with Canray Fontenot.)

"Clifton Chenier and his Red Hot Louisiana Band." Arhoolie 1078. (Essential recordings by the leader of post-war Zydico).

Haitian

"Divine Horseman: Voodoo Gods of Haiti." Lyrichord Records LLST341. (Classic field recordings of Haitian Voodoo ceremonies made by Maya Deren between 1947-1951.)

"Vodun Rada of Haiti." Folkways Records EFS-4491.

"Meringues and Folk Ballads of Haiti." Lyrichord Records LLST 7340. (Features field recordings made by Maya Deren of secular Haitian folk music.)

"La Troupe Makandal: A Trip to Voodoo." Gayrleen Records LP-1374. (Recent recordings of Voodoo ceremonial music performed by New York master drummer Frisner Augustin and La Troupe Makandal.)

Mexican

"*Sones Jarochos*—Music of Mexico Volume I." Recordings and annotated notes compiled by Dan Sheehy, Arhoolie Records 3008. (Traditional Jarochos music from southern Veracruz.)

"Lydia Mendoza—Texas-Mexican Border Music Volumes 15 and 16." Folklyric Records 9023 and 9024. (Early recordings of Mexican-American folk songs from the master of the tradition.)

"The First Women Duets (1930-1950), Texas-Mexican Border Music Volume 17." Folklyric Records 9035. (Classic Mexican-American ballad duets including selections by Lydia and Maria Mendoza, Juanita and Manuel Mendoza, Carmen and Laura, others.)

"A History of Border Music—Texas-Mexican Border Music, Volumes 1-19." Folklyric Records 9000 series. (Comprehensive survey of border music including Norteno accordion, mariachi and string bands, corridos (ballads), and other styles.)

Andes

"Mountain Music of Peru." Recordings and booklet compiled by John Cohen, Folkways Records ES-4539. (Includes field recordings of Amerindian vocal, flute, and string music.)

"Music of the Incas—Ayllu Sulca." Lyrichord Records LLST-7348. (Includes traditional Peruvian Indian music performed on harp, mandolin, violin, and flutes.)

"Perou: Taquile, ile du ciel. Musique Quechua du Lac Titicaca." Ocora Records 558651. (Includes field recordings of traditional Quechua vocal music accompanied by drums, flutes, and panpipes.)

"Charango Cuzqueno." Recordings and annotated notes compiled by Thomas Turino, Auvidis Records G 1504, 1985. (Features traditional Peruvian music by master charango player Julio Benavente Diaz.)

"Sounds of the Andes: Street Music of Cuzco, Peru." Recordings and annotated notes compiled by Bob Haddad, Lyrichord-7393. (Features traditional vocal music accompanied by harp and mandolin.)

For further information on folk and ethnic music recordings contact the following distributors:

Rounder Records
One Camp Street
Cambridge, MA 02140

Lyrichord Records
141 Perry St.
New York, NY 10014

Folkways Records
Birch Tree Group LTD
180 Alexander Street
Princeton, NJ 08540

Arhoolie Productions
Pablo Ave.
El Cerrito, CA 94530

Music of the World
P.O. Box 258
Brooklyn, NY 11209

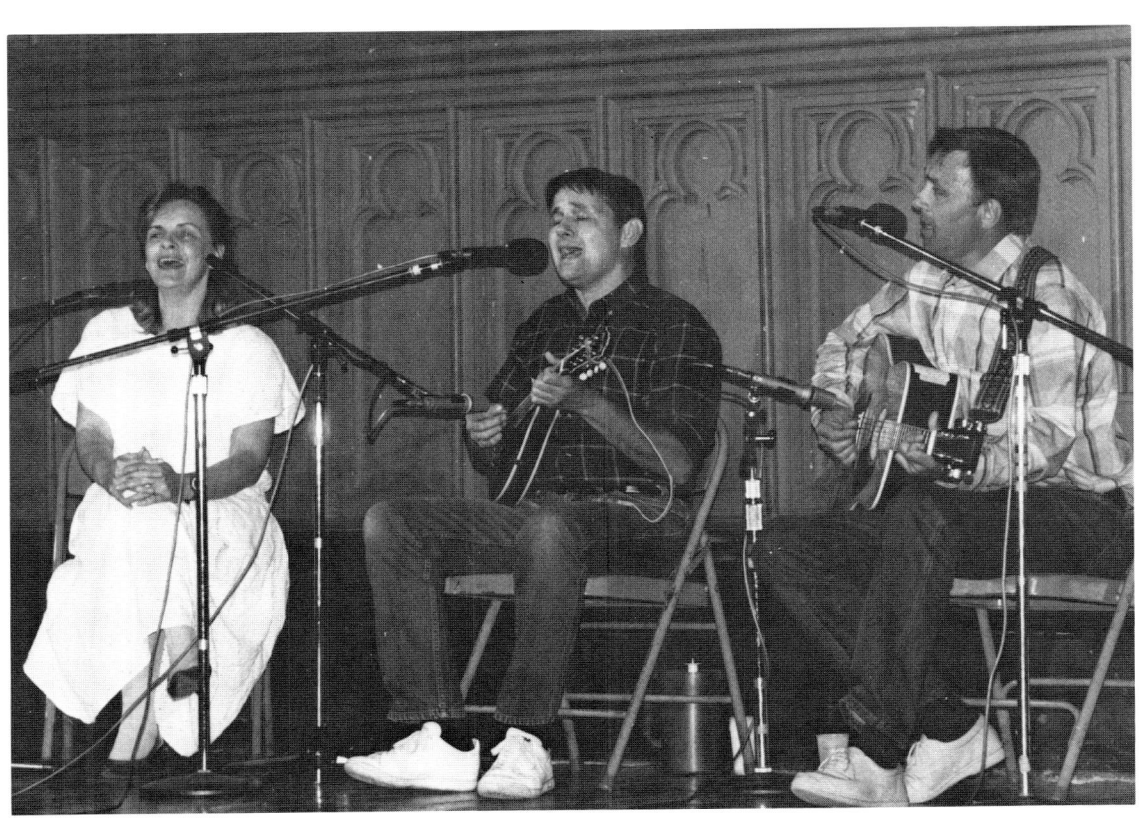

The Whitstein Brothers with Ida Whitstein.